Blooming Through
LOSS

Tending to Grief with the **BLOOMPATH**®

Eryn Elder, MA

Cover Design by Eric Labacz
Edited by Kate Allyson
Formatted by Tamara Cribley
Permissions by Mary Jo Slazak Courchesne

Permissions for cited material have been obtained by the respective copyright holders.

Paperback ISBN: 979-8-9928794-0-7
eBook ISBN: 979-8-9928794-2-1

For permission requests, please contact:
Roots and Wings Grief and Loss Coaching
eryn@rootsandwingsgriefcoaching.com

First Edition: April, 2025
Printed in the United States of America

Disclaimer:
This book is intended to share insights and offer support for those navigating grief and loss. It is not meant to replace professional medical, psychological, coaching, or therapeutic advice. If you need additional support, please reach out to a qualified professional.

A note about the examples in this book:

In this book, I share the stories of Lani, Jane, and Scott among other examples of individuals. While these stories may reflect the experiences of individuals I have had the honor to support, they are not drawn from actual client narratives. To honor the privacy and confidentiality of the individuals I work with, these examples are composites, drawing on insights from the many people I have encountered in the realm of grief and loss over the span of multiple years.

Keeping a journal nearby to capture your reflections as you read through this book can be a valuable tool for deeper insight and enhance your self-understanding and engagement with the book. There is a companion journal that you can get here https://www.rootsandwingsgriefcoaching.com/griefandlossbook.

If you find yourself feeling overwhelmed, trapped in despair, or struggling with depression, the guidance of a mental health professional can be invaluable. I encourage you to seek professional support when needed, as it can be a crucial step in your healing journey. I hope this book brings you renewed hope and guides you toward a deeper connection with your true self and purpose.

With warmth,
Eryn

Contents

Preface

"The act of blossoming requires vulnerability and courage, as
we shed our old layers and embrace new growth."

—Anonymous

Grief is a natural response to loss of any type and it affects many aspects of our lives. When grieving, we have both internal and external responses. Because of grief's taboo nature, friends and family may not understand how to support a griever. And yet, we all grieve. Bad things happen. We are conditioned to respond in a specific way until we break that cycle and realize what does (and does not) serve us.

This book has been a work of heart and mind, soul and inspiration. My daughter died unexpectedly ten years ago, and I have been grappling with what grief means ever since. I have always enjoyed writing, and I did not realize over the past ten years that this book would come to be until the BloomPath® started to form in my mind and being. Shortly after my daughter died, I was sitting outside in the Colorado sun with my sister. While the sun felt much too bright, I felt inspired to share about a new hope starting to form.

"What's next?" she asked.

"I need to write. Grief is an all-encompassing mystery that I wish I could help others and myself better understand and navigate with hope," I replied.

That was over ten years ago, and at that point in my grief, I knew I wanted to write, but it was not something that would happen quickly. I have had many doubts about my ability to make myself this vulnerable. And yet, if I can survive a loss as crippling as the death of my daughter, I hope I can write something that leaves a positive impact too.

Your grief does not need fixed, and you do not need cured. Your grief exists beyond your mind, and we do not know enough about grief to say that it is felt, internalized, thought about, or acted on in a specific way.

It is okay if you feel stuck. Or depressed. Frustrated. Full of anger as part of an emotional response to an injustice or bad thing. Our work as part of our grief is to turn that into something that serves ourselves and others. It is part of the meaning making we must do as we take what we learn in life and weave it into something filled with purpose and kindness.

If you are currently grieving, thinking you should be grieving, never grieved, or didn't grieve how you wanted to and needed to, felt alone and tired in your grief, or have done just fine and don't feel you need to grieve, this book is for you. It encourages you to take a holistic yet microscopic curiosity about your own grief and loss experiences, leading to new insights and new tools and strategies for meaning making, purposeful living, and enhanced ways of being.

If you are a friend of a griever, please take a moment to acknowledge the complexity of grief and all its touch points within and outside of someone. My hope is this book grows your compassion for the grievers in your life as they navigate the multifaceted and complex nature of grief. Be there for them, with their agenda, not yours. Ask curious questions from a place of non-judgment and for the individual's own learning, not yours, and stay out of judgement mode when you are with your friend who is grieving due to a loss.

Some losses take us to the depths of despair. Yet in the despair, there is hope. Once you know grief, you know its lowest points and its heights, which transcend your current way of being. And our way of being and thinking in the world needs to be examined and grown as we keep expanding our capacity for thinking and goodness.

This book is for adults—current grievers, past grievers, friends, family, companions, and caretakers of those dealing with loss, either current or past. While many of the activities in this book are directly for a griever, reading this book as someone who can help someone with loss is just as important. You may also discover grief that lives inside of you that you have not yet tended to, and now have a more purposeful opportunity to do so as you work through this book.

If you are in the early days and months after a loss, be gentle with yourself. Some of the activities may work better for you at a later time while others may be helpful now.

Wherever you are in your grief journey, please know that you are not doing it wrong. With some scaffolding and support, you have the tools within you to create a meaningful life filled with open heartedness and authenticity.

Hope in the Valley

They say life manifests peaks and valleys,
But that which should be nuanced,
Is the descent into the valley.

As a hiker knows,
Treading from peak to valley,
Takes time and is gradual—
You do not just fall from peak to valley.

But, in life, that is exactly how the descent goes.
I can be at the peak, or ascending, and without caution,
Tragedy strikes.

There is no acclimation to the valley.
I descend like a stone thrown in water,
Only swifter even,
Falling to a new depth unfelt before.

The valley swallows me.
Tears me apart, cradles me,
And re-purposes me,
With a surprising intentionality yet with a newfound lack of clarity.

As I emerge,
The soft tufts of grass provide some comfort,
Some place to land as I get back up,
Only to fall again.

But the valley is not bad after all.

It is where I am forever changed,
Maybe for the better.

I start to feel the ground under my feet.

I can look up and see a mountain peak in the distance.
There is hope and there is fear.
I cling to both, hoping that hope clings to me.

While the ascent may seem impossible,

I start to recognize that I can look up with hope
And see the climb may be gradual, it may be swift, but

That does not matter.

Because I will climb again, a vessel of new compassion from the valley.

I will get to know myself as I ascend and fall—
There is no up, or down, only the wisdom of here leading me, guiding me.

The journey of life is unknown—
I will ascend and descend uncharted paths,
changed this time,

Uncovering new perspectives, new joys, new hopes, and new life.

Chapter 1

Introduction to the BloomPath®

"Hope is available during grief and suffering."

—Anonymous

I wrote the Hope in the Valley poem about three years after the death of my daughter Evelyn Claire Elder, in response to the deep grief I was feeling. My first-born daughter died unexpectedly as an infant and was rushed to the local emergency room from her daycare and died from Sudden Unexplained Infant Death Syndrome (SUIDS[1]). She was such a light in our life. She was a beautiful baby with piercing blue eyes and full of contentment, especially fond of music. Prior to writing this poem, I could not access a pathway forward for coping with the strong emotions I had about the place where I spent my last days with my daughter, Breckenridge, Colorado. This poem was one outlet to help me create movement for my feelings to tend to them and gain new insights and finally to get back to a geographical location I loved.

After Evelyn's death, I switched careers to move into the world of grief care. Making the change into the grief profession was something I did not know would lay ahead of me for "new life." I had been working as an administrator of a coaching program at a university, and a few years later, left that work to stay home with my two living children. After spending the summer with my children and getting to know them in a new way, I launched into that fall with newfound creativity, spiritual renewal, and self-compassion. I was on a walk when grief and loss coaching as a career entered my being. I knew that my career in coaching crystallized in the form of grief care when every fiber of my being lit up, my arms got goosebumps and my mind ignited. At that moment, a new life began.

From my professional training in coaching, grief support, and master's in education, to the work I have done with grievers, to studying my own grief responses, I began to plant seeds for what I created in 2022: The BloomPath® for Grief and Loss.

This model goes beyond linear and singular approaches for grief support to a holistic, creative, and practical understanding of your own individualized grief and loss journey and helps you create your unique grief path with, through, and into the future. The book helps you understand how to apply the model to your own grief and loss experiences.

There are so many life events that create loss.

Loss can include death, divorce, pregnancy, job, home, pet, identity, health challenges, chronic conditions, and more. The Grief Recovery Method has identified over forty life experiences you may have that may cause grief[2]. Grief and loss are all around us, all the time, whether it is in the form of a previous loss, current, or a friend or family member's, or a societal experience (such as September 11 in the United States or COVID and its effects). Just as you tend to these losses cognitively, it is invaluable to tend to them wholly. No matter where you are in your grief, you are not doing grief wrong. My objective with this book is to give you a framework that you can use to increase your understanding of your grief and loss circumstances to gain more clarity about who you are and increase your self-belief to live a good and authentic life.

In the BloomPath®, there are thirteen Blooms. These are represented by the circles on the model. These Blooms are intertwined because they all interact with each other. The six on the inside are your internal Blooms and the seven on the outside are your external Blooms.

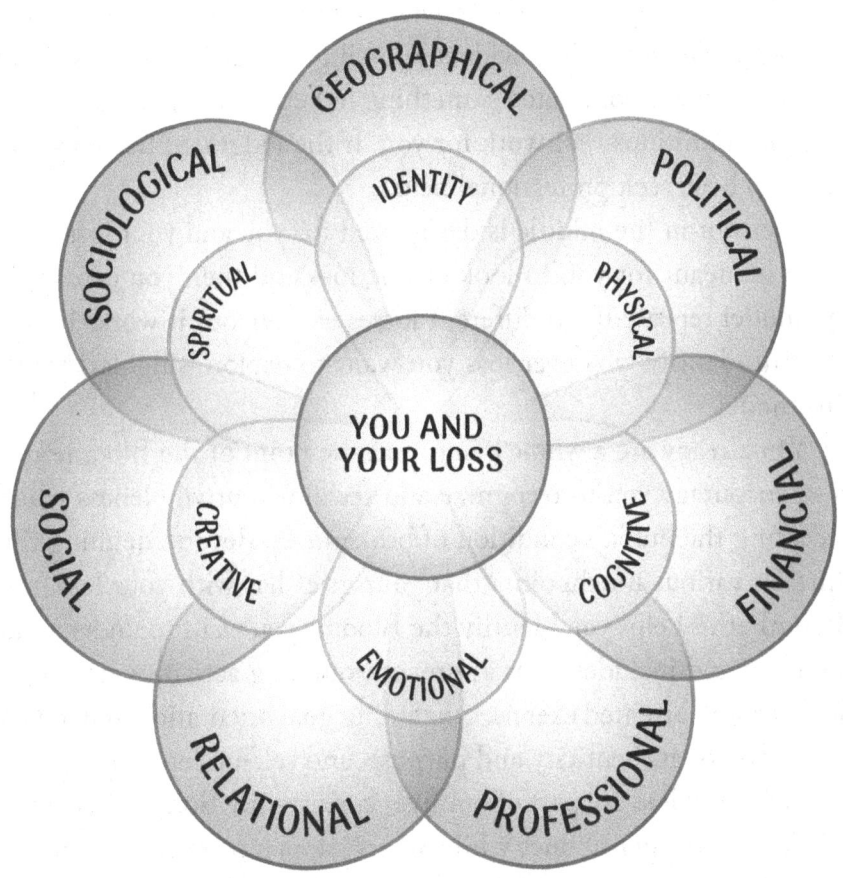

The circle in the middle is your root of you and your specific loss you are exploring with the BloomPath®. Outside of that are your internal and external Blooms where I have found that grief may have a touchpoint within your life. You want to be in a space where you can be curious about your reflections, trying to withhold judgmental thoughts about yourself as you embark on this type of reflective work. If those judgmental thoughts come up about yourself, try switching them to curiosities by asking a kind question about the judgment you are holding.

For example, someone may think, *"I do not have the willpower to try something new that will help me."* They can then switch this thought to a curiosity by asking, *"When did I complete a task that took five minutes and was helpful for me?"* This is evidence of willpower. Being curious about a time when you completed something to better understand yourself and the conditions that work for you. If the judgment becomes too much to bear, seek professional help.

The root in the middle is designated for you and your loss. This circle is meant for you to look at one loss and then you can apply the model repeatedly to different losses as well, but it works best if you can identify whatever loss you want to explore singularly with this model.

You already are a whole being, and the point of the BloomPath® is to encourage you to recognize and reclaim your wholeness while accepting the human condition of brokenness. Beyond defining the thirteen various touchpoints that your grief has with your loss, the BloomPath® helps you identify the Blooms you want to understand the most and includes clear awareness-building activities and hope-filled, action-oriented exercises including goal orientation, self-belief enrichments, authenticity and purpose, and self-understanding.

Grief and loss are part of our lives consistently. Sometimes many grief events happen at once while others happen years apart—no one has not met grief. Some of these experiences have larger impacts on us than others, and some losses go completely unacknowledged in our lives because of the busyness and lack of support to grieve them. For example, have you recently moved onto something in your life that is positive, and yet, have feelings of sadness? Me too. And so do many others. But, if you have the space and intentionality to grieve what you left behind, even if it was not particularly life-giving for you, you can process that loss so that you are freer to live more authentically and peacefully in your next life chapter.

On the other hand, what losses have necessitated the most obvious and robust grief for you? For me, it was the unexpected death of my daughter. It was not until that loss that I realized how inadequately I had grieved my other losses and life transitions. During the most intense times of grief, I tried so many different healing opportunities, which eventually led to the creation of the BloomPath®.

Grief and loss are so difficult to treat because it cannot be treated. It needs to be understood, and that looks different for everyone.

Having tried therapy, medication, acupuncture, groups, spiritual resources, and more, I realized I was missing my unique, individual compass—one's true self that guides us through difficult circumstances, but even it could use a bit of scaffolding, a bit of a pathway to support us through shifting beliefs and as part of our grief responses.

I am here in my personal grief and loss journey from my lived experiences as a teacher, writer, coach, researcher, mentor, leader, friend, family member, mother, spouse, and as me. After better understanding all these parts of myself through the BloomPath®, I now have more clarity about my own grief, and I revisit the model for my own grief care from time to time. Please join me on your personal journey with grief and loss by Blooming into your true self and finding solace and hope as a griever.

Part personal narrative, part workbook, part reflection, and filled with my honest observations on grief and loss after working with the grieving and experiencing grief, this book will provide you with personal honesty and best practices in grief care while providing you a new model to explore your grief and loss. The BloomPath® is a scaffolded guide to help you listen to yourself and the life-giving outside sources of strength and renewal for your new life. It is accessible, holistic, and practical for anyone at any place in their grief.

The BloomPath® is for anyone who wants to explore their grief and loss in an individualized and supportive method. Whether that is a life transition, a change of location, divorce, a death of a, pet, child, grandparent, grandchild, parent, sibling, or a loss of identity, a loss of use of physical abilities or mental abilities—grief is all around us. Grief is our response to loss, no matter how big or small. There is so much grief floating around our world that we need more conversations about grief and loss to help people process their grief in a way that is healthy and individualized for themselves that supports their well-being, their livelihood, their engagement with life, and what is to come after.

In each chapter, I include various stories and examples that are loosely based on those I have interacted with in the grief and loss space, along with my own experiences. Each chapter concludes with a reflective exercise. You can use the Grief and Loss BloomPath® over and over in your life circumstances and grief experiences because the model is responsive, adaptable, individualized, and accessible to work for you and whom you are and whom you are meant to be. You may tell the whole truth about who you are and what it is like to be you.

There are a few ways to apply the BloomPath®.

Imagery and metaphor may help us understand our life with more depth and compassion, and that is one of the reasons why I created a model that is filled with imagery and metaphor, and yet, is tangible. As you move through chapter two, you will learn about opening yourself up to your vulnerability to engage thoroughly with the model. I begin this next chapter by defining grief and sharing my personal narrative with grief to express my vulnerability so that you are welcome into a space to be vulnerable in your own reflections too. In chapter seven, I explain the paradox and its importance to your life and the work with the BloomPath®. I have defined the paradox as a way of understanding that shows up in grief and loss that shifts our world and causes us to relate to ourselves and to others in different and unexpected ways. Grief is the complexity of love, loss, and life. To grieve is to experience/hold the paradox of humanness that opens a new path filled with greater love.

If you are in the first few months and year of your grief experience, please hold yourself with care and know you are not alone. Take the time you need to listen to yourself and your wants and needs. Sometimes, all we can do is get out of bed, and other times, we may be working multiple hours a day and interacting with many different people. For some, they want and need to be more active in their grief, and for others, they need to slow down. Despite wherever you are, rest is important. You are okay wherever you are, and no one can judge you for that.

Grief is a root, and it opens you up to exploring other areas of your life that may need shifted, tended to, or felt more fully. By rooting into your grief, you open yourself up to transformation and a life that you want to live while honoring your loss.

Chapter 1 Exercise

Take out a journal and answer these questions:

- How do you define grief?

- What has been your experience with grief so far?

- What is your intention for reading this book?

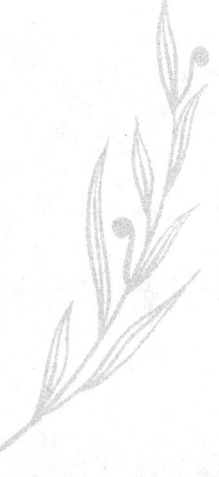

Chapter 2

The Roots of Grief

"We fear that grief will erase us. But, it is not erasure. It is transformation."

—Anonymous

Grief may be a response to any type of loss including death, divorce, pet loss, job loss, home loss, life transitions, identity shifts, or anything that you had attachment to that is no longer in its current form and/or relationship to you.

Grief affects many aspects of your life. Grief:

- creates complexity with your feelings and thoughts

- includes internal and external responses

- feels unnatural although it is a natural response to loss

- includes external systems and relationships.

Grief is not a one-time event. Compounded grief occurs when we experience many losses in an abbreviated time period. Compounded grief is also known as cumulative grief. Sometimes a singular grief event can lead to additional losses, and other times, people may face various losses that are unrelated over the course of a few months or years. Compounded grief may lead to difficulty coping or finding healing modalities that work for an individual because of the complexity of dealing with multiple, untended losses. With this compounding, it may feel more and more difficult to cope. But there is hope.

I was in despair for at least a year after the death of my daughter. It is nothing that can be escaped, and I tried to tend to it while also feeling completely unequipped to know what to do or how I should be grieving. I was grasping at my authenticity, not knowing how to act, and thought I needed to be in my grief all the time. I helped pass federal legislation, started a scholarship, planted a memory garden, planted a tree, journaled (briefly), attended therapy, played the piano, played volleyball, utilized support groups, panicked, slept a lot, tried multiple medications and sleep aids. I read self-help and spiritual texts, mostly from a Christian and Bahá'í lens, and didn't find anything overly adequate during those early months, although reading brought me comfort. I was trying to cure my grief rather than experience it.

Despite trying to find multiple modalities for healing, I finally realized that there really was nothing adequate when it came to grief because, as a culture, we do not support the griever, and we don't support grieving well. There needs to be more availability for others to witness your pain and for you to feel safe being witnessed in pain. Nobody wants others to watch them in pain, which is understandable. We want to protect both ourselves (from being vulnerable) and others from having to feel our pain. But if you cannot be vulnerable, cannot be yourself, it puts you in a very hard place. I have lived this despair.

New people come into your life in grief. From the new friends I made to the people who could stand beside me in my pain, I was fortunate to know many compassionate people as I grieved. Various neighbors, co-workers, a few family members, spiritual leaders, and peers drew me in when I could not give something back. They generously gave their time and companionship amidst the complex lives they were living.

A few months into my grief I was so shaken, confused, paranoid, and depressed, I asked my husband, Matt, to go to the police station to get the police report about the death of my daughter because I was certain that there was something undisclosed in there pointing to me. This moment was scary for both of us. I was spiraling in shame and guilt. And Matt was grappling with his grief in his own way. I did not have the strength to access the report, and I know this was far from pleasant for him to do, which made me feel more shameful and sorrier that I asked him to do something so painful.

Matt read the report, and I thought that would ease some of my pain. It did not. With the wonky sleep schedule from being a new mom and the terror of the reality of losing my first-born daughter, I just could not shake that Evelyn's death was my fault. My shame and guilt enveloped me, and I lost myself. That is when despair set in, and I entered the abyss. I smelled smoke and thought that I would finally end up in jail or prison as I thought I needed to be. That's where I thought I deserved to be. This grew out of the fact that I felt like I could not be vulnerable in my pain.

And the reality is—most people do not know how to accompany people in their pain: they want to fix it, they want you to move on very quickly, they want you to stop hurting, and they also don't want to feel the pain. Before Evelyn's death, I held this mindset too. People have good intentions, but they do not want to know that you are now broken (even though you were broken before) because it may cause them to acknowledge their own brokenness and pain. Through the grief that I experienced, I realized that being broken is a part of everyone's journey, and it was time for me to really grow into that and absorb what that meant, embrace it and Bloom from it. I was not quite to that understanding in my thinking at the time. I was still in the place believing, truly deep-down believing, that I belonged in terrible places. I know I have done broken things in my life that I've learned hard lessons from. In that moment in my grief, those all came to the forefront of my being, so I was only able to recall all of my faults and bad decisions. These and the complications of the world weighed on me in a current that pulled me under, lacking the porousness and buoyancy needed to stay afloat. Nobody belongs in those spaces of despair, and yet, that space brought me on a new path that was so much better than my prior way of being.

I heard from a few people this would make me stronger, which was unhelpful. I needed a space to fall apart and land safely. Everybody deserves the opportunity to heal in a place that provides support and understanding. I was on my way to finding out what that level of support looked like for me individually because I let go of the rope holding me from falling deeper into the well and landed at the bottom.

I ended up at a mental health hospital during this time where I was diagnosed with a major depressive disorder that included a psychotic break, which happens when depression becomes too much to bear. I experienced paranoia; I thought the police were after me for the death of my daughter. This was my first time dealing with the mental health system as a patient, and I was prescribed medication that would help me sleep and get my sleep back on schedule, still grappling with Evelyn's loss in addition to my post-partum hormonal shifts too.

Evelyn died in the throes of me being a new mom. I had been waking up extra early to breastfeed, and suddenly everything switched. I went from a fractured sleep schedule where I was caring for Evelyn, to abruptly not caring for another human life, though my body was signaling to do so everyday all day. I felt like I had all the time to sleep in the world, yet I was wide awake all the time. The mental health hospitalization was not glamorous. The sterility was coupled with prison imagery, and yet, I found my footing.

At that point, I was so depressed that I literally fulfilled that metaphor of once you hit bottom you can at least kick your feet off the bottom to come back up again. I had fallen apart beyond what I knew I was capable of, and I lost control of my being. The darkness, though, is what lets the light in and brings hope and meaning, as painful as it is. So, I surrendered a bit more to receptivity and found an inner strength to kick off the bottom and let myself and others pull me up. Radical honesty liberates the soul, and I began to explore what that level of honesty meant for me.

That experience helped me realize how difficult it is to grieve as a human. This vulnerability grew my compassion for others and gave me a break from feeling like I needed to be strong and self-sufficient and that I could lean into my sensitivity with more intention and purposeful healing. While the hospital was not ideal and not where I wanted to be, it gave me a landing pad for myself to face my biggest fear that Evelyn's death was my fault and to explore my guilt, which weighed so heavily on my soul. This part of my journey opened me up to new possibilities for what life can be when approached from a place of less judgment and more authenticity.

I had just turned twenty-nine at the time, and I was still finding my way as a young adult after graduate school and figuring out who I was now that I had lost my daughter and had willingly left my job. Leaving my job created another heavy grieving event for myself because I had wrapped so much into my career identity that I had lost a lot of myself. I thought that the more educated I could become, the higher-level career I could have, that I would have what I wanted and needed. I would find myself, my authenticity, through my career, and that was so inauthentic to who I am and untrue for me. Education and learning were important to me and my career, but I needed a way to integrate that into my life where I did not anchor into my career for my identity. I learned to anchor into myself, and I find things that I love inside of me and things that I find difficult to navigate within me too. And I know this brokenness allows me to be more broken open, more open-hearted, more authentic, and supportive to not only myself but those around me as well.

Compounded grief is often part of your grief and loss journey and can happen at any age. As people grow older and become caretakers of their parents or others, compounded grief may be experienced as we enter a phase of life where we start to lose friends, siblings, parents, pets, jobs, and more. Essentially, this is a stage of life where compounded grief may show up consistently among grievers in relationship to both death and non-death losses. I also have known many incredible young humans who have dealt with compounded grief at a young age, too.

If you are dealing with compounded grief, there is hope. As an adult, you hold wisdom at this stage of life that you did not hold earlier, so you can root into the hopeful moments of that wisdom to support you as you grieve multiple losses and change how you want to respond.

What does compounded grief look like? Let me tell you about Lani. Just six months after her mother died, Lani's dad was diagnosed with cancer and then her marriage started falling apart. Lani did not have much time to grieve the loss of her mom, when so many other losses started to manifest. Her relationship with her mom was steady, so when her mom died, she felt both anger and hope—anger that she did not get to say the things she really wanted to say to her mom and hope that she could find her way through this, having grieved the death of a friend many years ago.

She remembered that talking to others helped her in her prior grief, so she scheduled a few grief support meetings. While this met some of her needs, she realized that this grief felt a lot different than other grief. She went to her partner to express her needs, and she felt stifled. She needed more rest, more support, more care, and she struggled to find outlets for these needs. After a few months, she started to feel a bit more whole again, spending time with friends and engaging with her work. Then, her dad was diagnosed with a progressive, stage-four cancer, and she felt at sea again, not knowing how she would get through supporting her dad as his main caretaker and being a wife, worker, friend, and more.

The more Lani provided care to her dad, the more she wept about the loss of her mom. She knew how much of a rock her mom was for her dad, and she knew her mom would be a more effective care-taker than her. She started to doubt herself more and tried pouring herself into her work and caretaking duties. She found that she and her husband started becoming more distant, and she was exhausted by the end of the day. She would fall asleep un-showered and full of dread and sadness. She needed to know where the care for her was as she worked through each day, exhausted. She began to seek understanding about her loss experiences in her life. Lani's story continues later in the book.

While I provide a roadmap to use the BloomPath® through this book, it may also be helpful to take some time to work through the BloomPath® in a way that is authentic to you. You already are a whole being and broken being, just like all other humans, and the point of the BloomPath® is to encourage you to recognize and reclaim your wholeness while accepting the human condition of brokenness.

Chapter 2 Exercise

Think about the losses you have experienced over a brief period of time, possibly a few months to a couple of years.

What were they? Include any type of loss that comes to mind.

- How did each loss affect how you felt about the last?

- Which loss impacted your other losses the most?

- Which loss do you want to further explore that you have not yet tended to in your grief?

- How does this reflection help you tell your story?

Chapter 3

The Five Roots of Grief Support

"Sometimes it takes only one act of kindness and caring to change a person's life."

—Jackie Chan

Care needs to happen in the early parts of grief and is not to be forgotten in the years after. Caring for yourself is necessary both in the early parts of grief and in the weeks, months, and years following. When you care for yourself, you are doing whatever you need to do to ensure you are safe and healthy while being gentle with yourself for mistakes and missteps. There is no exact formula for supporting someone and yourself in the early days and months after a significant loss. Being stuck is okay, and the rest of the book activities may flow more easily later in your grief journey. However, you may want to start on these activities sooner, and that is okay too. Wherever you are is okay, even if it does not match your local culture at the time or even the expectations you have for yourself. But in that darkness, the roots begin to grow.

I developed this model because I struggled tremendously in the first few months after the death of my daughter. I wanted and needed care. I wanted to love myself but could not find a way to be okay with where I was at in my grief journey. In reflecting on the five roots of grief in this chapter, I benefited from some of them but did not have access to the others yet in my grief process in the early months after my loss. I include the five-part model for you to consider the Blooms in the BloomPath® and how you may receive care, be open to receiving care, and to care for yourself amidst the heartbreak and challenges of reorienting to yourself and the world around you. Consider how the Blooms fit into these roots of grief and look for moments of hope within each of these parts.

My neighbor Astrid would stop by regularly, and about a month after my loss, I was not doing well. "I think we just need to sit here for a moment and scream aloud together," she said when she stopped by to see how I was doing after Evelyn's death.

We screamed as loud as we could. The scream was healing. She let me be seen by her being vulnerable too. Her compassion and ability to sit with me in the difficult space from a place of non-judgment helped my healing. This was early on in my grief journey after the death of Evelyn and is an example of care. Since that interaction, I have reflected about what may be especially helpful and accessible to people early on in their grief experience.

As I continued to learn more about grief, I kept revisiting the idea of a model for support for early grievers that may also be applied at any time in your grief and loss.

The blog post ideas for my website naturally flowed from both my professional and personal stories. As I wrote more posts and engaged with the work of grief and loss support more fully, a five-part grief care model began to emerge, grounded in best practices in grief care and my understanding of how to best support those dealing with loss. This model synthesizes information in the book and serves as an additional pathway for hope and healing. While it may be especially helpful for those early on in their grief journey, it may be used as a supportive resource for many years out from a grief and loss experience too. There are five roots of grief support: care, resources, network, emotional curiosity, and receptivity.

I developed this model when I noticed many people wanted something that they could easily share with themselves and with others to support their healing as they grieved or as they supported an individual going through grief and loss. Later in the book, I include activities to engage with the BloomPath® through intentional goal-setting activities and reflections that help you go more in-depth with your self-understanding and individual wants and needs. For some early on in their grief, possibly a few days to a few months after the loss, it may be helpful to start with the five-part model for early grievers. This model can be applied at any time in grief and loss, and fits into the BloomPath® too.

The Five Roots of Grief works for both the griever and those supporting someone grieving, so take a moment to consider how each of these parts may integrate into your own grief care and care for others. Each of the following elements can be reinforced with your reflections regarding your internal and external Blooms. Parts one, four, and five may more easily relate to your internal Blooms and two and three to your external Blooms explored in the following chapters. Select what works best for you.

Care

Explore how you show others care and show yourself care. Care consists of acts we show ourselves that put our wellbeing at the forefront of our priorities. It also includes how you nurture your thoughts to show yourself compassion and how you engage the spectrum of your emotions and way of being for healing. What works for you when you show yourself care? What does not help you care for yourself? How can you include the type of care that works for you more frequently throughout your days, especially your more challenging days? For example, as a friend or family member of a griever, check-in on the individual with opportunities for connection such as invites to take a walk or to drop off tea. Two women who were my neighbors cared for me this way, and it meant so much to not be so alone. Try finding ways to stay connected or start to connect with others whom you feel emotionally safe with and can be yourself. If you are grieving, is there someone you can reach out to who will relate to you with care? Focus first on the Internal Blooms—identity, physical, cognitive, emotional, creative, and spiritual—as you continue to find ways to care for yourself.

Resources

Consider how you access the resources you need. Resources can include mental health or coaching support as well as spiritual and physical health support. Check out what is specifically available to you in your local communities. Are you feeling lonely and want to find connection? What resources can help you? Look for local support groups, online support groups, neighbors, friends, and/or family. On the other hand, do you need a break, and if so, what resources can support your need for some time and space? For example, I heard from a man how he tried various support groups after the loss of his child, and they were not quite the resource he needed. He then tried a new exercise option and wrote about his feelings, and talked about how hard this process was to find the right resources for him. Recognize it may take time finding the best resources for you, so try to stick with finding what you need.

Network

How do you engage with your network? Your network includes the people around you from personal to professional relationships; those you work with to the family and friends who can support you as well as individuals you have encountered in earlier parts of your life and those who are now coming into your life as a result of your loss. What help can you ask of your network? For instance, is there a simple adjustment to your seating at work that would make things more comfortable for you to have the privacy you may need to grieve throughout the day? Or, for example, do you know your friend enjoys organizing things, and you could use her support getting your home organized? One individual said they wanted help with cleaning their home and another with laundry, but neither wanted the same help as the other. Everyone needs and wants different support, so let the griever know how you can specifically help them, and then, they can say yes or no. For the griever, it is hard during a vulnerable time to know what you need and to ask for what you need. Try to be bold by asking for what you need or having someone help you ask for what you need. It often feels like you do not now what you need, and that is okay. Try to embrace the smallest things that you may want to try or need and ask for them. For both parts two and three (resources and network) you may benefit from focusing specifically on the social, relational, and sociological Blooms as you find the care that you need.

Emotional Curiosity

Part four focuses mostly on the Emotional Bloom from a space of curiosity. For part four, how can you ask yourself questions about how you are doing and what you need from yourself? From others? How are you noticing your thoughts? Feelings? Here's a short exercise for noticing and feeling your emotions:

1. Take a few, slow deep breaths and notice your thoughts and feelings and internal changes such as heart rate.

2. Tend to your feelings such as by simply observing them and naming them or being curious about them without judgment.

I have heard from various individuals about their frustrations with themselves for either feeling too much or too little. One woman noted that she does not feel her emotions, so it was difficult at first to do this exercise. However, once she had a chance to really sit with the words that described her feelings, she went from stuffing her feelings to understanding them better.

As you continue with the book, you can hold this framework to help you engage more fully with the exercises in the BloomPath®.

Receptivity

Acceptance is a word that comes up a lot in grief and loss. It is even in the Stages of Grief[3]. People want to know how they can accept a loss. Various aspects of a loss may not always be accepted, though, and that is okay. Focus on receptivity rather than acceptance. Receptivity is the willingness to consider or accept new suggestions and ideas. We can be reflective about how we move through transitions in relationship to our grief and loss when we consider resistance. The opposite of resistance is acceptance or receptivity. I like the word receptivity much more than acceptance. I can relate this to my own grief and struggles with acceptance regarding various aspects of my daughter's death. I do not necessarily have to focus on acceptance; rather, I can be open to new and more hopeful pathways for my future and lean into my becoming. Sometimes when we focus on acceptance too much, we get stuck and try to force ourselves into thinking or feeling a certain way about our loss, when we just simply cannot. Receptivity allows for this and opens you up to new possibilities while holding space for your grief. Consider how receptive you are to what you are noticing about yourself and what is unfolding now.

Chapter 3 Exercise

Think about where you are in your grief journey and answer these questions:

- Which of the five roots—care, resources, network, emotional curiosity, and receptivity—do you feel most supported by in your grief experience?

- Which root do you feel is least supported?

- Which of the five do you typically do best when helping others? How can you apply that same level of care to yourself?

- Which Blooms stand out to you the most in relationship to The Five Roots?

Chapter 4

Expanding Your Roots

"Grief is a journey, not a destination."

—Anonymous

Losses impact other losses. From the un-tended parts of our grief from previous losses to the similarities and differences between losses, it can be easy to tangle up our experiences, thoughts, and feelings, which may impact how you grieve a current loss and how you live in the years after loss.

One exercise in particular can help you expand your understanding about your losses and help you reflect on your relationships within a singular loss that may have the most unfinished business in your life, so that you have more clarity about your wants and needs.

This is a strategy that I learned while enrolled in the Grief Support Specialist Course, from the University of Wisconsin, known as a Loss Complexity Graph. This graph exercise is based on content from the Grief Recovery Handbook/Grief Recovery Method and is an example of one that Lani used to explore her losses. She listed her losses from left to right with the left being the most impactful then to least impactful with the years they occurred. After that, she shaded the loss that has the most unfinished business—note in her example, her most impactful loss and the one with the most unfinished business are different. That is often the case, which helps draw attention to this discrepancy.

Example of Loss Intensity Graph from Lani's Story

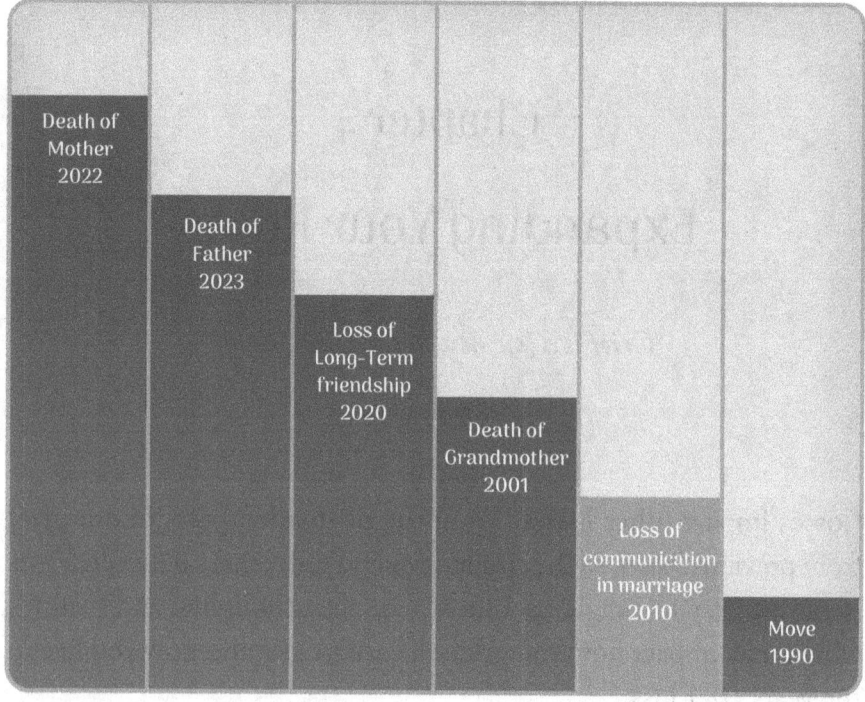

By writing about both the positive and negative aspects of your shaded loss, you can begin to tend to that particular loss that may be impacting your current loss or the loss you have explored throughout the book. This particular loss may be tended to by writing about it, seeking out a therapist or coach to discover more about this loss, or using movement as a strategy to process the loss, or revisiting strategies throughout this book. You may also want to compare these graphs with the BloomPath® to discern how you want to address the loss. Here is an example from Lani's graph where she mapped her positive and negative moments that resulted from her identified loss.

Positive moments: Loss of Communication in Marital Relationship

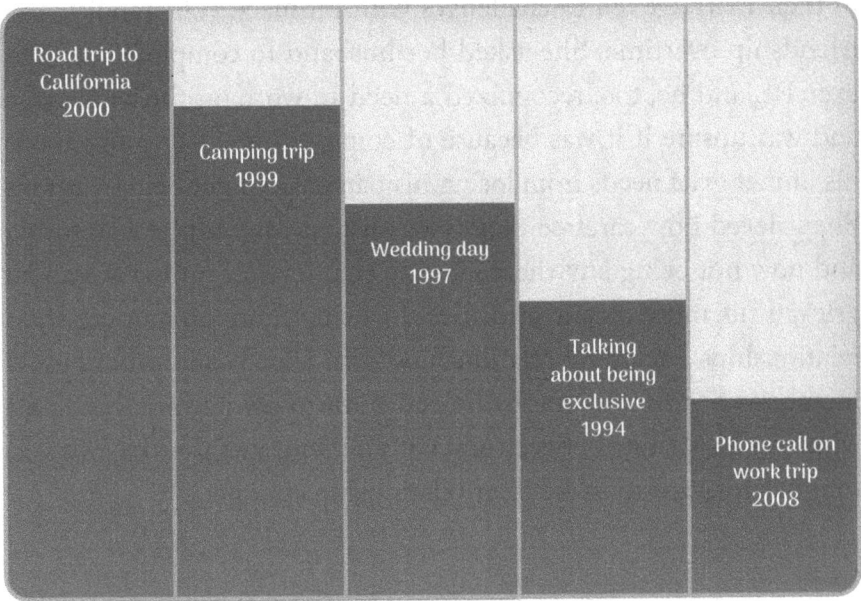

Negative moments: Loss of Communication in Marital Relationship

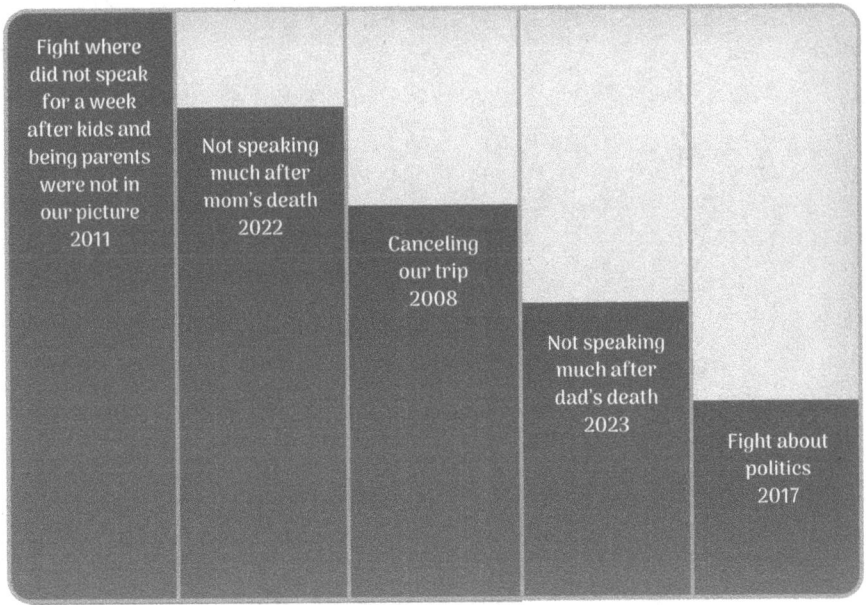

As Lani completed the Loss Complexity Exercise, she became increasingly aware about how the lack of effective communication in their marriage led to challenges with intimacy, vulnerability, and friendship overtime. She asked her husband to complete a similar exercise, and he, too, recognized a need to work on their marriage and was unsure if it was because of communication or more about his unmet grief needs from losing his parents and not being a parent. She grieved how carefree they were on that road trip to California and now not being anywhere close to that level of intimacy, and he grieved his more recent priorities, focusing more on gaming than relationships, including relationships with friends and other family members. Seeing the graphs helped both to gain awareness about what was happening between and within them, and how they wanted to move forward to make their relationship stronger.

Chapter 4 Exercise

Complete the loss complexity exercise. Start with the **Loss Intensity Graph Instructions**.

1. Brain dump all of the losses in your life that come to your mind. Go back and add in years.

2. Order the losses from most significant to least, and include a brief title of the loss and the year(s) it happened.

3. Create a bar graph with the most significant loss on the left and the least significant loss on the right.

4. Keep doing this until you've entered all of your losses or relation-ships into the graph.

5. On your loss intensity graph, shade the loss with the most unfinished business. This is the loss that you intuitively feel the most pulled to heal. This shaded loss is the one you will prioritize for this exercise.

If you prefer a more writing-centered exercise as an alternative to using this graph process, you can write a few paragraphs describing your losses and relationships to those losses after you complete your brain dump of your losses.

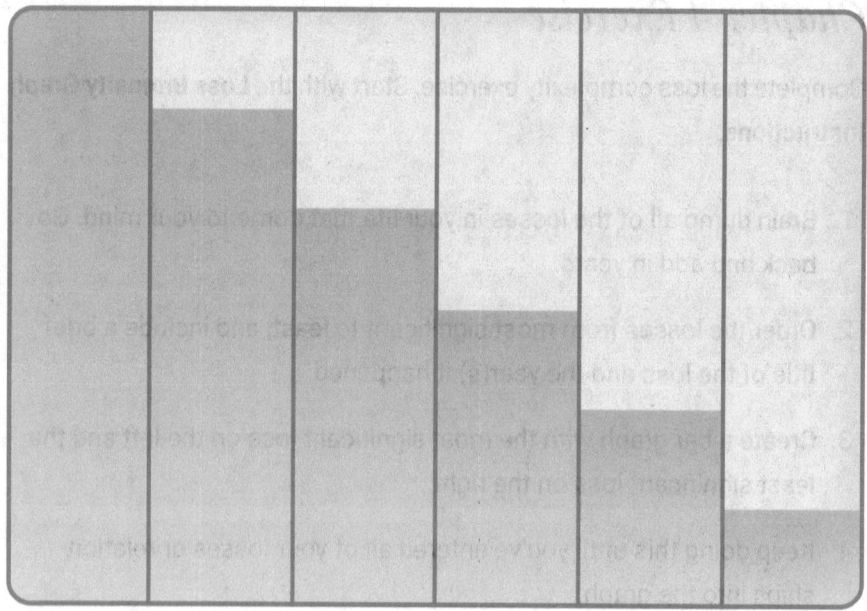

Relationship Complexity Steps

1. With the shaded loss, brainstorm positive and negative moments related to the loss, the relationship you had with the person or thing.

2. Create two separate bar graph charts with positive and negative moments, where they are listed from most impactful to least impactful.

By writing about both the positive and negative aspects of your shaded loss, you can begin to engage with tending to that particular loss that may be impacting your current loss. This particular loss may be tended to by writing about it, seeking out a therapist or coach to discover more about this loss, or using movement as a strategy to process the loss, for example. You may also want to compare these graphs with the BloomPath® to discern how you want to address the loss and grieve as you need to do so.

Positive moments:

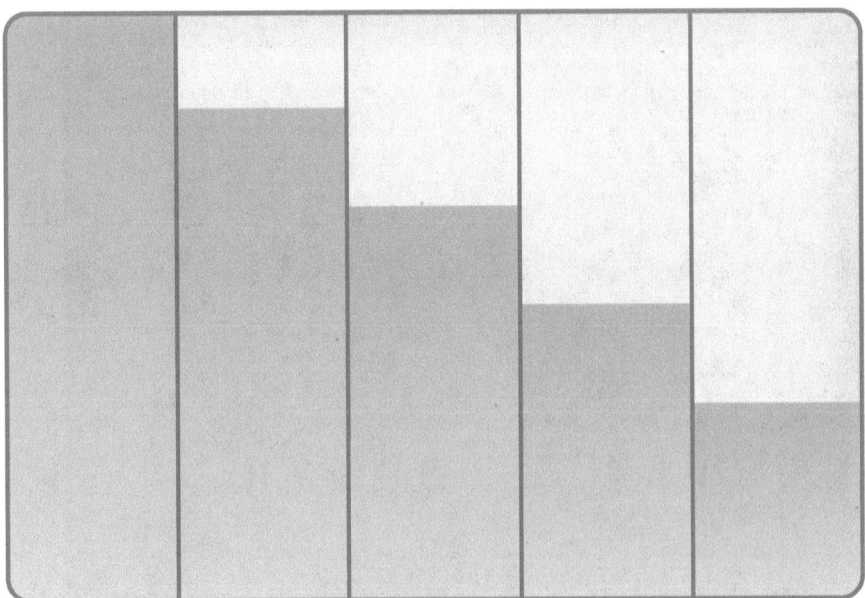

Negative moments:

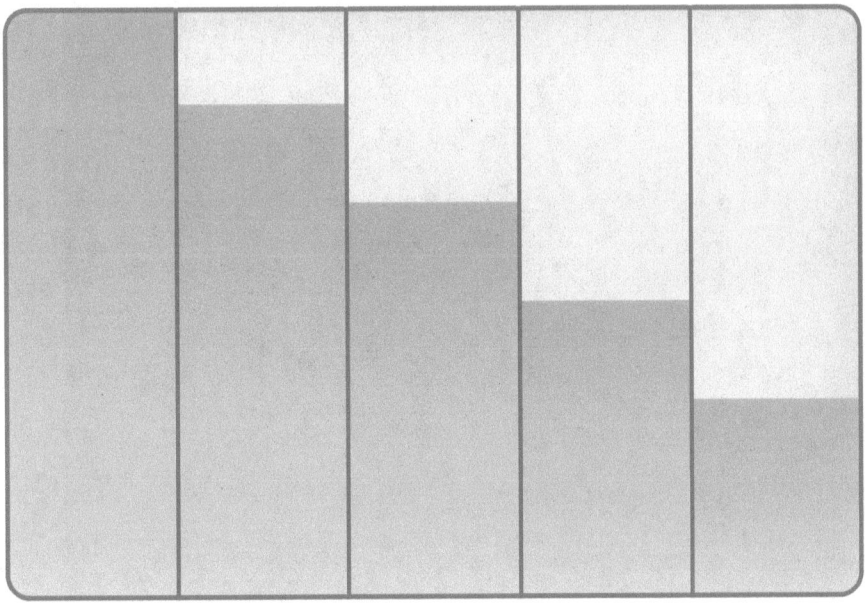

Chapter 5

Cultivating Roots

"Grief can be the garden of compassion. If you keep your heart open through everything, your pain can become your greatest ally in your life's search for love and wisdom."

—Rumi

You carry your grief with you. When tended to, your grief may be integrated into your life for authenticity and hope. In the early months of my grief and loss, I struggled with tending to my grief with compassion and care. You have opportunities to tend to your grief in a kinder way if you have not yet done so. You can feel the pain of grief while being compassionate to yourself. And there will be external factors that affect your grief. You are not alone in navigating these challenges. Seek support and continue trying resources until you find something that brings even a microscopic light into your life. Also, it can be challenging to discern the difference between grief and a potentially diagnosable mental health challenge, trauma, and/or other health concerns. The complexity of grief is profound and navigating grief with all these compounding factors may require extra support, and that is okay. You do not need to be perfect to love yourself; remember to love your past self and love your future, wiser self. Hold your current self with that same love.

You can use the BloomPath® to explore multifaceted areas of your life to create movement. You may gain new insights to become the person whom you are meant to be, whom you want to be. The BloomPath® can help you understand the roots of your being and the wings of the flower that allow you to change and grow and Bloom. You will root into your grief, loss, and yourself, into whatever philosophies or spiritual frameworks work for you. You can use your grief to gain hope to live a good life, find more meaning, and understand yourself more, so you can integrate your grief into your life.

In the past, professionals thought you grieve and move on, and grief really was not a part of you after that initial mourning and grieving period. Now we know that is not true. There are so many myths about grief[4]. The myths I built up in my own mind in the early months after the death of my daughter were that no one understood. I could not be vulnerable with anyone because people were constantly judging me. I believed I had to be suffering all day every day or else I wasn't grieving, and I needed to hold onto my pain and suffering to stay connected to my daughter.

While there may have been kernels of truth within each of these myths, they were not wholly true, and I needed to find ways to navigate that nuanced space—to be okay with my anger regarding judgment toward me and to hold space for grace. I could honor my daughter by taking moments for contentment and happiness too.

One other factor of the BloomPath® for Grief and Loss is that it allows you to revisit those facets of your life that are myths about your grief as you encounter new grief and as you continue to deal and grapple with older grief experiences.

Tending to this type of hurt is a lot different than healing a broken bone. While writing this book, I was in a car accident where I severely broke my wrist, and it had shattered into multiple pieces, and I had to undergo two surgeries. I had four different substantial incisions (and now scars), to make my wrist whole again. At the most basic level, a broken bone simply heals when treated. Yes, both grief and a bone need deliberate healing, and both need time to be left alone. However, when the broken bone is healed, you can use it again, possibly with some level of adjustment, but you don't have to revisit that type of break in a way that you need to revisit the broken heartedness of grief and loss. My broken bone is not as extensive as the breaking I had in grief.

The breaking in grief is what lets both our light in, and our biggest challenges open into something more beautiful. I did not experience this level of breaking open to possibilities when I broke my bone. I grieved my running schedule, and playing the piano, and lifting things, but I was easily able to adapt and find strategies that worked for me. Simply put, grieving my broken bone and the car accident was just much easier for me. Additionally, people now see my external scars and ask what happened with such concern, and I appreciate the care. On the other hand, the scars of grief and loss are often unseen, so people do not relate to those with the same level of concern as they do with the scars they can see. We do not have to see what is in front of us to have compassion for ourselves and others.

The tending of grief and loss is much more nuanced and complex, and the healing continues to change as you change. A bone is going to stay a bone. You are not. You are an individual who is gathering and amassing multiple lived events that only you hold, and therefore, your whole being is constantly in a state of healing and change. Your time spent with your grief is deep work. It is not something you have to do all the time. In fact, it is invaluable to give yourself breaks from it. But you need to tend to it when it shows up and treat yourself with care and kindness.

Here you can start to plant your understanding of the Blooms and how they relate to you. The BloomPath® contains thirteen Blooms. Six Blooms are focused on the internal aspects of your life, and seven are focused on the parts of your life where grief and loss may have multiple touchpoints in your life. The six Internal Blooms are: identity, physical, cognitive, emotional, spiritual, and creative. These Blooms all focus on the inner aspects of your life. They are part of who you are.

Internal Blooms

The Identity Bloom includes your gender, sex, economic status, ethnicity, abilities and disabilities, culture, and anything else that uniquely defines your identity such as your values. All of these are part of the Social Identity Wheel[5]. Questions of identity often come up in grief and loss, and part of the work of the Identity Bloom is to better understand your traits and culture.

The Physical Bloom is where you consider everything regarding your physical self, including your eating habits, sexual health, physical health, sleep habits, and relationships with your healthcare team. Physical health is separate from the Emotional and the Cognitive Blooms so that you can distill within each of these Blooms where you might be needing more support, keeping in mind these Blooms are intertwined with each other.

The Cognitive Bloom describes the thoughts you are having about your grief and loss, including your mental processes and the effects of grief on your brain. In short, we know grief impacts our brain, and our brain searches for ways to create a new map in grief, which is challenging because of the dissonance this creates[6]. This Bloom also includes your thoughts, logic, philosophies, and beliefs about your grief and loss as well as your daily task management. Grief may open you up to thinking about new ways of being and new ways of thinking about yourself and the world around you.

The Emotional Bloom includes how your emotions are affecting you internally and externally. Your emotions affect your thoughts, behaviors, and actions. Notice how your feelings show up for you in your mind, body, and behaviors.

The Creative Bloom includes any creative outlet you have or have used for your grief such as music, art, writing, journaling, comedy, or poetry. This also provides space to explore how your hobbies are being impacted by your grief and how you are relating to your hobbies as a griever.

The Spiritual Bloom includes various facets of your relationship to a higher presence which could or could not include church or other places of worship, spiritual readings, nature, meditation, your own intuition, some may say their soul, and others are unsure. In grief and loss, individuals may further explore questions of spirituality in direct relationships to their thoughts and emotions that they are experiencing. These grief experiences often bring up thoughts and feelings that draw us closer to a spiritual source or further away. When I explored my spirituality with more intention, it became a vital source of renewal and inspiration.

External Blooms

There are seven external Blooms: geographical, political, financial, professional, relational, social, and sociological.

The Geographical Bloom is your actual physical location. This includes everything from your relationship to the land and where you are located and the natural world that surrounds you to your housing, the rooms within your home, and even the photos on your walls. This Bloom is of particular interest to me because of the nuance related to the physical geography and the natural geography and how they are both wrapped up within the grieving journey. Additionally, where you are located in the world also impacts your grieving experience due to how grief is normalized or talked about in your geographical area as well as what resources are available to you for supporting your grief journey.

The Political Bloom also impacts your grief and loss and can often be overlooked in grief. You have your societal and moral beliefs, possibly party affiliations, and you participate in political movements that may or may not relate directly to your grief and loss but have ancillary effects on your grief journey.

The Financial Bloom represents the resources, income, investments, the broader economy, and general economic stability that can also be a part of your grief and loss. Grief may have a financial impact, either positive or negative, on you, and navigating these changes on top of the other changes you may be encountering as part of your grief may be difficult.

The Professional Bloom includes your work and your professional identity which includes your current career, prior career path, future possible career paths, your jobs, and your unpaid work, including work done in the home. Because many of us are in these workspaces more than most other spaces, grief is inextricably tied to your work. I received the phone call about my daughter's death while I was driving home from work, so I had to do a lot of reflection about my work and how that related to my grief. This overlapped with my identity work in the Identity Bloom, and I had to untangle my values, wants, needs, and perspectives about how I relate to the concept of work.

The Relational Bloom includes your close partner, family, and/ or your close friend relationships—people you talk to regularly and whom you can rely on. These relationships may impact your grief and loss, and this helps you explore any changes you need to address with your immediate relationships as you navigate the grief and loss process.

The Social Bloom includes your connections with friends and family who are more acquaintances and may not fit in the Relational Bloom. These are people that you might see in the workplace rather frequently or are people whom you have known in your life for a while but have not stayed overly connected to. This also includes your social media, and how, when, and what you utilize social media for and how that relates to your grief and loss.

The Sociological Bloom includes various institutions and their relationship to you as an individual, your family, and your grief and loss. These institutions may include the education system, medical system, government, healthcare, economic system, and family systems. This Bloom helps you inquire about the systems you are situated within and how they support or challenge your ability to grieve authentically. Historically, many of these systems have created inequities in accessing quality grief support, and too many voices have been left out of these systems. The many truths about grief and loss have been lost due to the masking of these voices.

I have found that grief may have a touchpoint with each of these thirteen Blooms, and that is why I have untangled them in this BloomPath®, so that you can explore what you want and need more freely and with more intention—gaining a greater understanding of where and how you want to focus your grief support needs. When we can untangle part of the messiness of grief, we can tend to it more specifically, confronting our own needs and desires, as they are changing in response to our new understandings and learnings from grief.

I have collaborated with various individuals in their grief as they have explored this model, and overwhelmingly they have responded to this model differently, including which Blooms they choose to explore and how they engage with them. In this book, you will be guided through a few intentional ways to work with the Blooms for your own healing.

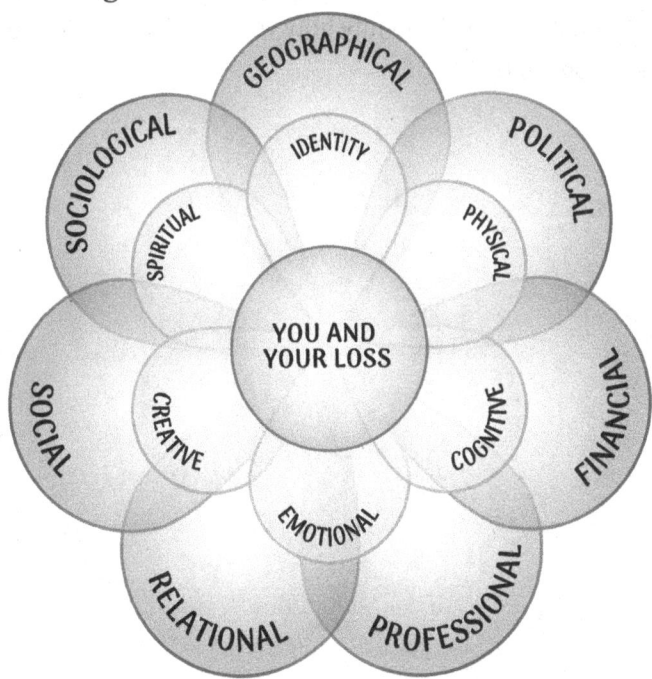

Chapter 5 Exercise

- Before exploring the Blooms, take a moment to reflect on the descriptions for each of the thirteen Blooms. What stood out to you? Why? Was it something related to experiences, or relationships, or your own internal thoughts and feelings? Take a moment to journal your initial responses to these questions.

- Reflect on the descriptions for each of the Blooms. Add in additional descriptors, thoughts, and feelings for Blooms that stand out to you.

- Choose a loss to explore in the book using the BloomPath®, possibly the loss from the Loss Complexity Exercise in Chapter Four or a loss that is now coming to mind for you. The loss can be any type of loss, and here are a few examples: death loss, divorce, job loss, home loss, pet loss, identity changes, belief changes, a life transition. At a general level, identify how your grief relates to the Blooms in the BloomPath®.

Chapter 6

Watering Roots

*"There is messiness in learning to love yourself after
loss. There is beauty in the process you engage to re
enter the world both changed and unchanged."*

– An observation from the author

"Ever since my mother died, I feel like the light in my candle went
out," Lani told me. She was still grieving the loss of her mother while
dealing with her father's cancer and her relationship problems that
were introduced in Chapter Two.

This is an effective metaphor for what happens physiologically to
our bodies, minds, and spirit when we are grieving a loss.

Some used to think that we would have a few difficult feelings
to navigate, to integrate into our lives, and that we would miss what
we lost and that is it. That was grief. We know grief is so much more.
With the neuroscience of grief and loss we recognize that something
physiological is happening in our minds in addition to our internal
processes and external relationships. It makes sense that we are dazed,
distracted, and confused, and our bodies may need more rest while
grieving. The energy that grief consumes is unseen energy, so if you
are constantly tired, please be gentle with yourself. There is no formula
for how much rest you need in grief, but this need typically shifts, so
listen to your inner voice. Additionally, your mind creates a new map
in its own brain structure when going through grief. In the book *The
Grieving Brain*, Mary-Frances O'Connor explains that you may need

to allow your brain to have experiences day after day while grieving, which updates the brain to orient to a new map[7]. This may help you relearn your world and create a level of buoyancy in your grief. Rest and experiences can go hand in hand.

Coupling this physiological understanding with the multi-faceted Blooms, you can now take moments to understand your development through grief: who you are, who you want to be, where you are in your life, what you feel, what you think. This is all going to be quite different for everyone. Some may feel like Lani, losing her candlelight, and others may feel that some type of candlelight is burning brighter in them, accessing more intense emotions or feeling a renewed sense of purpose. Some may feel all these feelings at once, while others may be feeling numb. And, these feelings may shift within a day, over a series of days, weeks, months, and even years. Those feelings will continue to shift, and you can create meaning from them using the BloomPath® in whatever way feels most helpful. These reflections and your exploration with the BloomPath® help you create meaningful experiences to update your mind-map and understand yourself more.

Now that you have an introduction to the Blooms and a model for support, you can discover your grief needs utilizing the BloomPath® in different ways. The BloomPath® will help you reflect on your wants and needs regarding your grief and losses. The BloomPath® also helps you acknowledge and discover the areas of strength and difficulty in your grief and loss.

One way to use this model is first to create more open awareness by journaling responses to the questions I am including in the following chapters for each of the Blooms. These are questions to help you get started in your reflection process. Feel free to use other questions and follow your own thinking and feelings. This will help create movement for where you want to explore and make shifts regarding your experience with grief.

During my grieving process early on, a woman in a SIDS[8] support group sent me a journal specifically for those who were grieving a child loss. When I received that journal, I felt numb. A few journal prompts resonated with me, but nothing really helped me to write, and I did not do a lot of journaling at that point, and that is okay. Writing was not necessarily a healing modality for me in those early months. And yet, I wonder if I had more scaffolding with the questions I was trying to respond to in my own life and a model that accompanied them, I may have journaled more. The prompts were one sentence prompts with questions such as write about your day. The journal questions were one every few pages, and I could not find a way into or through writing about them because of the ambiguity of the responses I yielded, my numbness, and the lack of scaffolding. You do not need to force yourself into a practice that is not working for you. As you explore the questions, take time to consider multiple things that may work for you, and keep what is working and discard what is not.

Revisiting Lani's story introduced earlier on in the book, a few more months passed, and her dad's treatment was working. She saw a new life in her dad that also gave her hope, but her sadness about her mom did not subside. She and her husband started to have more heated conversations about how they were spending time, and while they used to have time in the evenings to connect and watch television or play a game, now, she was going straight to bed, and he was immersing himself in video games. His grief for his mother-in-law was complex since their relationship was no more of that than an acquaintance, and his communication skills were not overly effective, especially in higher-stress situations. He lost his parents when he was much younger, and he never received grief support. He preferred to deal with loss by moving on, which is what he learned to do when he was younger. Their gap in grieving modalities and understanding each other's needs began to increase. The stress of their marriage challenges started to take a toll, and instead of a day between conversations, it turned into a few days, and then weeks.

Because her dad started to show signs of improvement, she focused her efforts more on her marital relationship. They decided they would work on their communication by being more vulnerable with each other about how they were feeling and what they were thinking and taking the time to talk through challenges. They took a few weekend trips, and they started to grow closer again.

As they grew closer, her dad's health declined, and at the end of the year, he died. She felt both the weight of guilt for feeling like she did not do enough and the tinge of reprieve believing he was no longer suffering. She was angry that there was not a more efficacious cancer treatment for her dad. She started to have complicated feelings about her mother's death again. Guilt regarding unexplored elements of her relationship, and a deeper loneliness and sadness than she had felt before. She had a much more robust goodbye for her dad's declining health, and she began to have overwhelming feelings of guilt and sadness about her mom's death.

She started to feel the familiarity of not really being able to open up and ask for support from her husband that she needed because her feelings were a bit different this time, and he struggled with his communication. As a result, she felt like she had to do and hold so much but did not have the energy. She wanted to invest more time in her relationship. She did not want to tell her spouse how to support her because she wanted to be around people who would intuitively understand how to support her. She started to feel guilty about unexplored elements of her relationship with her husband, and he did not know how to respond to her grief, so she began isolating herself more at home while attending support groups in the community and seeking online support too.

Lani realized that she was most ambivalent about her social relationships from the BloomPath®. Not able to open up and ask for support from her husband in the way that she needed because her feelings were different this time, and her husband's communication skills were still lacking. She felt like she had to do and hold so much but did not have the energy. She wanted to invest more time in her relationship. She tended not to reach out to friends when she needed support, which is a role she enjoyed playing in relationships. She realized she wanted this support from friends but did not know how to access it. She spent time talking about rooting into a few old relationships and growing the relationships in her online support group. As she stumbled through awkward conversations, she noticed that she had a lot in common with a woman in her support group, so she found the courage to set up a coffee chat. Lani's story continues in future chapters growing her roots and opening her Blooms for continued healing and hope.

As you reflect on your own story, my hope with having the broad availability of the questions that will follow is that you might be able to reflect on them and journal if you can. If you are not in that space, that is okay. Sometimes it may be challenging for a griever to focus on writing and reflection, which is why I scaffold understanding each of the Blooms with questions to help you consider their relationship to your needs. The way you explore them may be through writing, contemplation, conversation with others, or something else.

This is not a reflection that is meant to be done quickly, and it may take more time to go through some of these questions later, weeks and months down the road. I encourage you to read the questions and come back to them when you are ready to journal or process about them. You may also decide you want to draw about them, or create art or poetry about them, or reflect about them—it does not have to be only journaling. It may be helpful to even record yourself talking about these questions so you can go back and listen and learn where you may want to begin exploring the Blooms in the model. You can also discuss them with a close friend or therapist.

Take one Bloom at a time, just as if you were watering each of the roots, noticing what comes up for you with each Bloom. You may find that one or two resonate with you most or many resonate all at once.

Revisit Chapter Five that includes the descriptions about each of the Blooms. Reflect on those descriptions as you contemplate the questions about the Blooms in the following chapters.

As you work through the reflection exercise in this chapter, move to the Bloom that you feel most ambiguous about. Ambiguity is a challenging feeling because when you have confusion about something in your life, it can be particularly difficult to untangle both the ambiguity and your goals to tend to your needs. When you can explore your ambiguity about something, you create greater insight for yourself, which helps you set more meaningful expectations for yourself. Understanding what part of you wants to try something and what part of you is hesitant about trying that same thing may be complicated. For some, you may get stuck in the contemplation phase of making a change, and for others, you may decide a change is not right for you. And for some, you may jump in to making a change. There is not a "right way." Take your time and pay attention to both your wants and needs.

Each of the Bloom reflection exercises includes questions for you to consider and seeds of thought that relate to each of the Blooms. These seeds of thought are meant to give an additional nugget of wisdom as you explore the questions for each Bloom.

Chapter 6 Exercise

1-1-1 Exercise

- Circle the Bloom you want to explore in your grief the most.

- Square the Bloom you feel most hopeful about as a griever.

- Put a star next to the Bloom you have the least clarity or ambiguity regarding your wants and needs.

Why did you choose these Blooms? Stay curious about why you chose these as you read about each of the Blooms in the following two chapters.

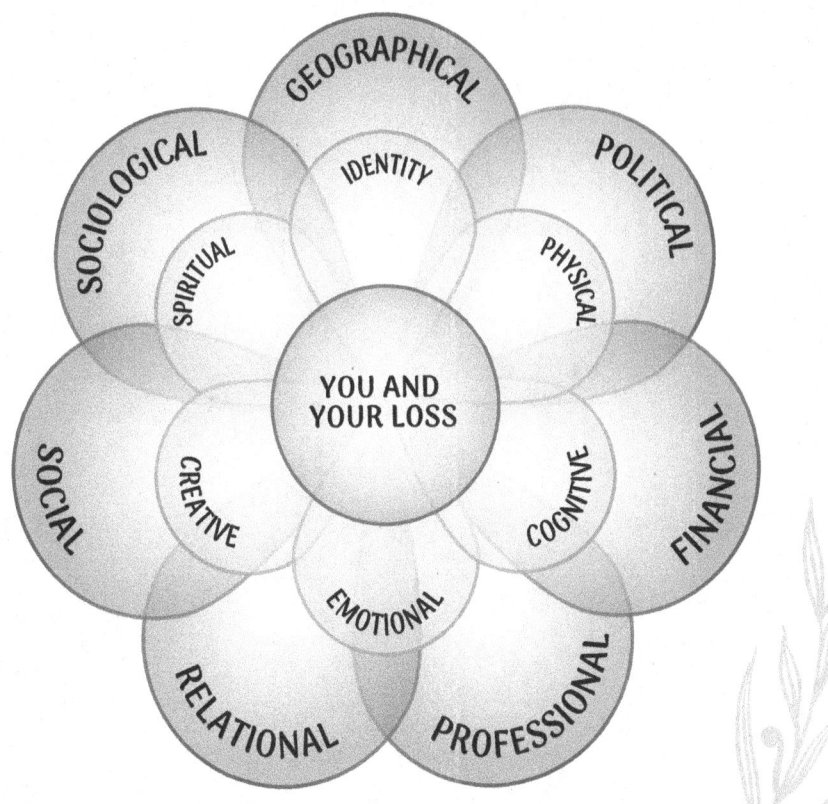

Chapter 7

Developing Internal Blooms

"The more space you give yourself to express your real thoughts and feelings, the more your wisdom will emerge."[9]

—Marianne Williamson

Throughout this chapter, there are reflections about each of the internal Blooms and questions for you to consider. As you read the reflections, pay attention to what comes up for you. Stay curious about the questions that create the most space for you to explore your grief and loss and who you are. You do not need to answer every question; these are here to get you thinking about each Bloom.

Identity Bloom

Who am I? Who was I? Who am I now? These are some of the pivotal questions that come up when exploring your identity in relationship to a grief and loss experience. Identity covers so much. So many people I meet say they were clinging to false identities prior to their grief, often because of societal or familial expectations. For me, I grappled with the question as to whether I was a mom and what that looked like after my first-born daughter died. My identity had been wrapped up in being a breast-feeding mom, and I asked the doctors to help me stop my milk production because I did not want to feel that break in my emotional connection with my daughter while grieving.

I had to consider who I was now—I did not know how to answer this question. Anytime anyone would ask me how many kids I have, for the first few years after her death, I would always let them know about my daughter Evelyn who died. Then, I stopped that approach because I became more aware of others and just wanted to talk less about what happened. And yet, so many people constantly ask that question, "How many kids do you have?" I still struggle with that question today, and I will either say, "I have three kids, two who are living," or "I have two kids." I still strongly dislike that second response, but it gets me by the awkward social interactions. So, who am I? I am a mother to three kids.

Our identities help or hinder our ability to access care that fits our individual needs. Find ways to cope with how your grief is intersecting with each of your identities. For instance, someone who identifies as male may feel that they cannot express their emotions of sadness because of societal standards. You may now be wondering who you are and how that relates to your culture. To help you, here are some questions you can ask about the Identity Bloom:

- Who are you?

- How do each of these identity factors influence your grieving process: gender, sex, ethnicity, socioeconomic status, disabilities/abilities?

- What are visible identities and invisible identities that you hold?

- What has shifted about your identity?

- What about your culture and values relates to your grief? How has this been helpful and/or challenging?

Physical Bloom

A few months after the loss of a child, a man was experiencing pain in his body. He went to his primary care doctor, and they did not find anything to pursue for medical treatment. He tried various modalities of exercise, stretching, walking, and still, felt these pains in his body. However, once the man accepted the impact of his grief, he began to fill his being with more self-compassion and that shifted things inside of his body, and he was not feeling his pain as strongly. Taking the time to engage in your grief from a personal development lens is not a replacement for traditional medicine. They complement each other. We are just beginning to understand how grief feels in the body, which makes it so hard to pinpoint the most effective treatment and healing options for physical medical needs and grief needs and their intersection.

The combination of various healing modalities has the potential to improve the quality of life for someone who is grieving. Some people I know have found healing modalities, such as sound bathing, float tanks, yoga, and energy work, to be tools for exploring their healing more fully, while others have found these outlets not as helpful. And even for some, they have revisited them at different times in their journey and realized new hope. These modalities often not only focus on the Physical Bloom but also on the Cognitive, Spiritual, and Emotional Blooms too. Use care when exploring these healing modalities, and let your care team know what you are accessing for healing support.

Your sexual health is often impacted. Grief may disrupt sexual intimacy, and it may play a helpful role in grief too[10]. Because of its complexity, it can be helpful to talk with a trained therapist about your sexual health. If you are partnered in a relationship, keep your communication about sex open with your partner. Grief likely has impacts, whether you lost your partner or have zero energy for sex while grieving a loss, or you are finding relief and growing intimacy through sex, hold yourself with compassion and grace as you navigate the complexities of sexual health in grief and loss, especially if you are mourning a partner loss. Try to be open about your thoughts and feelings about your sexual health.

Grief may impact other aspects of your physical health. Sometimes our sleep becomes disrupted, and that can be incredibly challenging. Other times, we may be getting just the right amount of sleep and then asking ourselves if we are grieving enough. Try to give yourself a break from judging whether you are grieving enough or feeling panicked about your new sleep situation. This may be true for other aspects of your health as well: your appetite, level of energy, etc. Some questions you can ask about the Physical Bloom include:

- How has your sleep changed/stayed the same?

- What is your relationship with food or other indulgences?

- How has grief impacted your sexual health?

- What healing modalities have you tried? What has worked and what has not?

- What healthy habits are supporting you right now?

Cognitive Bloom

The Cognitive Bloom is your thoughts about your grief. From the neurological side, your brain is shifting without a clear picture. I spoke with a woman in her sixties, Susan, about the experience of the loss of her husband on her cognitive functioning. She explained that when she went to the grocery store, she could not even remember what was written on her grocery list in front of her. From simple tasks, such as grocery lists, to more complex tasks such as interrogating your own thinking about your grief and loss, many cognitive aspects of your life may be impacted. And, in fact, many people that I have met tend to cry at the grocery store after loss. For Susan, we discussed ways to make simple tasks easier to provide more space for the complex cognitive task of grieving. Also, often reflections and questions such as, *"I used to think this about the world and now I think this. I am sure this thinking will subside, right?"* come up. This is a testament to the changes your brain goes through.

Your mind creates a new map in its own brain structure when going through grief. As mentioned earlier in the book, in the book *The Grieving Brain*, Mary-Frances O'Connor explains that you may need to allow your brain to have experiences day after day while grieving, which updates the brain to orient to a new map[11]. Questions you can ask yourself to explore the Cognitive Bloom include:

- How do your thoughts inform your emotions and/or behaviors?

- How has your worldview changed because of grief?

- What thoughts are now dissonant with your beliefs?

- What may help you feel supported to complete your day-to-day tasks?

Emotional Bloom

Some people have told me they are too numb to feel, and others say they are feeling too much. Our emotions can be all over the place in grief and loss, and we may even feel emotions we have never felt before at any point in our grief journey. I met with a man who said he was constantly crying. Some people cry a lot in grief, some a little, and some none. Some feel anger at varying levels, while others may notice their anger feels more like frustration or confusion. There are many, many emotions beyond sadness and anger too, some may include, for example: guilt, fear, despair, relief, confusion, compassion, gratitude, love, and more. These may be felt simultaneously, or you may vacillate between many emotions, including ones that are not congruent with each other.

We are different, and the emotional processes are not linear, and the range of emotions we feel may look different between people. If crying constantly is impacting your quality of life and you want to address that, then it makes sense to tap into your emotions to understand what all the tears are about and how they can be used as a source of healing and inspiration. On the other hand, sometimes we need to feel the spectrum of typically less-accessed emotions to break free from past traumas and ways of being that no longer serve your new life. For example, one low-risk healing modality if you are struggling with anger is finding physical ways to express anger, such as through Rage Rooms or exercise (for example martial arts). Emotions are an important part of our grief and losses, and we need to feel them to tend to them and respond in ways that promote your individual needs and goodness in the world.

Untangling our emotions, thoughts, and how we respond to these can be a powerful tool for navigating your grief. Understanding how you are feeling and what strategy you may want to try to tend to your feelings is important in your grief journey. Here are some questions to ask:

- What do you need to process your emotions?

- How are your thoughts impacting your emotions?

- How are your emotions impacting your thoughts?

- How are your emotions impacting your behaviors?

- How do you honor your emotions in relationship to your loss?

Creative Bloom

The Creative Bloom is often explored through hobbies, which tend to be creative outlets for many people. I once met with an individual who I'll call John. John found that he did not have the energy for his prior hobbies. At the same time, he wanted to find something to process his loss besides therapy. Painting became an outlet for him. He expressed himself with this modality until he had more energy to pursue tennis again.

Comedy can also be an outlet for grief; however, it can also feel inaccessible. Improv comedy and other forms of comedy have been helpful healing modalities for some while others have found painting or learning to play an instrument helpful. And for many, it is a mix of various creative modalities.

Sometimes we have moments of enhanced creativity and sometimes we struggle to access our creativity in our grief. At the same time, some of our tried-and-true hobbies may not work for us and sometimes they do. It is okay to try new things and go back to hobbies and creative outlets that are working for you now.

- What creative outlets do you enjoy (music, art, photography, poetry, etc.)?

- What songs, artwork, poems, etc. have held meaning to you in your grief?

- What is something you would like to explore about your creativity?

- What hobbies help you process your grief? Which do not?

Spiritual Bloom

"I always thought I believed in the natural order of the world until my child died." With my shifting beliefs about the world, I needed to root into various spiritual practices, including Christianity, Bahá'í, Hinduism, and more. Spiritual texts were grounding and comforting during this time. But, when people said this was all part of God's plan, it caused me to move further away from my spiritual beliefs, deconstruct them, and then find meaning in them again. Grief may cause someone to look at their spiritual beliefs in a new way. Give yourself time and patience as you reflect on your spirituality and what it is showing you in your grief. This may offer a comforting effect as you explore your grief and loss. Questions you can ask about the Spiritual Bloom include:

- How is your spirituality informing your grieving?

- What do you want to change about your spiritual practice? What do you want to stay the same?

- What religion(s) or beliefs inform your values?

- How are you relating to your spiritual needs?

Chapter 7 Exercise

Choose one of the Blooms from this chapter. Is this a Bloom you noted from the Chapter Six exercise? Journal or reflect on the questions asked about that Bloom in this chapter. Are there any other questions that come up related to that Bloom? In reflecting on that Bloom, does it lead you to reflect on any other Blooms?

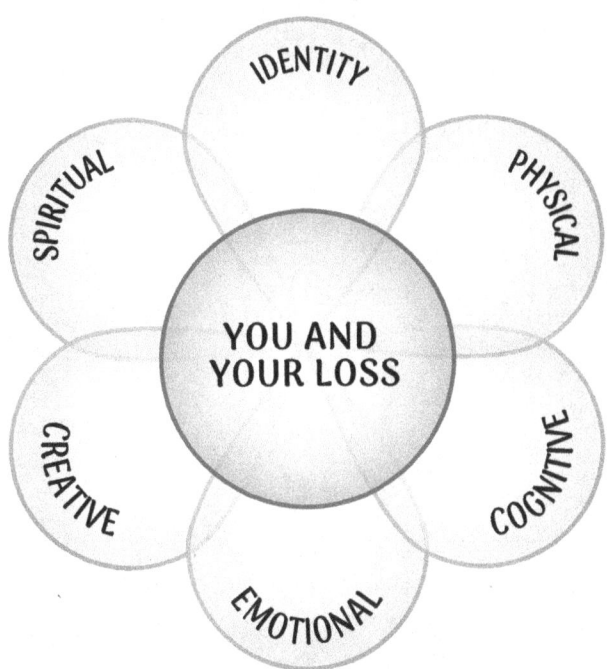

Chapter 8

Developing External Blooms

"Only when we are brave enough to explore the darkness
will we discover the infinite power of our own light."

—Brené Brown

Continuing with the development of each of the Blooms, let's now explore the external Blooms in more detail. Carry your reflections with you from the previous chapters to integrate your thinking and feeling about each of the Blooms.

Geographical Bloom

I spoke with a woman who said she just cannot grieve at all how she wants to because of where she is located in the world. Geography can impact our grief from the physical landscape to the cultural geographical landscape. She was constantly being judged for anything she did because it was not necessarily in line with the culture where she lived, and she did not feel safe disclosing to anyone in the community how she was really doing and how she felt. She rooted into the Geographical Bloom and realized that she could not physically move, at least not for a while, but she could do two things. First, she did a future visioning exercise to find a physical community where she could feel comfortable. Second, she looked for community outside of her geographical area to immediately find connection through various online options.

Sometimes it may be helpful to adjust your photos on your walls, and other times it may not be. If you try something to adjust the comfort of your home, and it is not working for you, feel free to change it again. Sometimes certain locations, such as grocery stores, may bring up emotions. That is okay to feel them wherever you are. Additionally, if you have recently moved and have not established community or roots, it may be helpful to seek out community-based resources to connect with others in the community. Here are some questions you can ask about the Geographical Bloom:

- How does your location impact your grieving process?

- What is your relationship with the natural world around you?

- What is your relationship with your home and its contents?

- How long have you been in your home and how does that timeline relate to your grief?

Political Bloom

So many losses are political. When my daughter died of SUIDS, I was heartbroken. And tried to do a lot of meaning-making. It was clear to me that so much more could have been achieved in politics to protect babies and toddlers as well as invest in understanding what happens to a healthy infant who suddenly dies in their sleep. Evelyn died August 19th, 2014. In November of that year, I flew out to D.C. to join Laura Crandall with the SUDC Foundation. She had been spear-heading the initiative to get legislation passed to have better data collection from the coroner's offices across the U.S. to streamline what they do and how they report in these cases. I participated in a fly in where multiple people from across the country met with legislators and their staff to help get the Sudden Unexplained Death Data Awareness Enhancement Act[12] passed under the Obama administration. This legislation streamlined how those who conduct autopsies store their data and improved how data is collected in all types of sudden unexplained infant death cases, as well as sudden unexplained death in childhood cases, which will be imperative to keep moving the research in this area forward.

Grief intersects with politics, and that is hard. You may have judgment around you about how you are grieving that is directly tied to the political ideological spectrum. You may be noticing how politics is showing up in grief, while those around you are not. Questions you can ask about the Political Bloom include:

- What political issues relate to your grief experience?

- How do your political beliefs inform your grief?

- What is the political landscape around you and its relationship to grief?

- What changing political beliefs are coming up for you, if any?

Financial Bloom

"I need help. I do not know what to do now that I have lost my partner. I need to find a higher-paying job and I want to honor the grief that I am experiencing now. I do not have the energy to find a new job right now." Someone may need to look at their current resources and discern if they have anything they can sell that would provide a bit of a buffer. What communities are you a part of? Who can help you within those? The financial situation may shift with a loss, depending on the type of loss you are navigating, and your relationship with money may change according to new values you are living out and how you now think and feel about money. Reach out to resources and support. Resources may include the ones you currently have access to such as friends and/or family. You may need to be bold and ask for extensions on payments and deadlines or actively seek community resources—as much as possible, rely on your network to help you if you are struggling.

When it comes to grief, you may need to be more open to financial support to access services that may cost money and/or look to your employer for employee benefits for health care, such as counseling, and bereavement leave or time off.

- How has grief impacted your financial health?

- What are your financial needs to be able to grieve in an effective way for you?

- How is this loss impacting your finances?

- What can you do to gain additional resources? Who can help you?

Professional Bloom

Career shifts come up all the time in grief and loss. Sometimes, it is because of a loss of a job or professional ability. Are you moving into a new role, staying where you are, looking for less responsibilities at work, or feeling inspired to take on more? So many things to consider regarding your professional life after a loss. One individual wanted to explore what it would take to leave the workforce, receive new training, and start a new job. Their motivation stemmed directly from their loss. They decided that they wanted to look for a lower-level job and work there while they developed the skills and resources needed to shift careers. This was a multi-year process tapping into authenticity and purpose. As part of the process of transitioning, assessments may provide a nice starting place as you discover more about yourself.

If your workplace culture does not have a grief aware culture, it is not your job to immediately change that. Rather, focus on your individual needs, and talk with someone whom you have a good relationship with at work about what you may need in the workplace environment while you grieve. These conversations at work may be challenging because of the complexity of the emotions and thoughts you are holding regarding your grief, and your potential impacted sleep, so take your time with these conversations. Ask others for help with wording communications or write out your needs and how they relate to work.

- Do you have what you need from work to grieve?

- What are your work policies for loss and grieving?

- What tasks at work can you do, and which ones do you need help with as you grieve?

- Are you in a career that is suitable to you after your loss?

Relational Bloom

"Ugh, I am so frustrated that I am not getting the family support I want and need," a woman told me. Our closest relationships can be a point of consternation or hope as we grieve. Some people are simply better than others at supporting grievers. As a griever, you want your friend, family member, or partner to know how you need to be supported and to be there for you in that way. The reality is, we may gently need to let others know what we need in our grief because of the lack of grief education in our culture and the shame associated with talking about grief. This is vulnerable and hard to do, and this is something that I did not do well early on in my grief.

Sometimes we may need to cut ties, at least for a while, and other times, we need to be vulnerable and let others know exactly how we need to be supported. Please note if you are supporting a griever, be curious about their needs and wants and forgo your agenda, following the rule of treating others how they want to be treated. Ask the griever what they need by giving options. For example, "Do you want to go on a walk, or can I help you with a task you need help with, such as communicating with your employer or bringing you a meal?" Affirm to them that it is okay that they are feeling however they are feeling right now. As a close friend or family member, it may be worthwhile to help the griever scaffold their supports to how they are feeling. For example, "I noticed you are sad. I do not want to fix your sadness, and I want to offer support for you in your sadness. Would a walk help or is it more helpful to you to sit with what you are feeling right now?"

Relationships are hard, regardless of grief. Be gentle with yourself as you navigate familial and close friend relationships. Some of these individuals are more empathetic than others. As the person grieving, you get to choose what is supporting your grief needs and what is not with these relationships. At the same time, if trying to navigate difficult conversations with family and friends is not working for you, take a break and find other outlets for support.

- How is your relationship with your family?

- What do you need from your family and friends?

- How do you communicate your needs to family and friends?

- What is supportive from these people? What is not?

Social Bloom

The individual was feeling very disconnected, having struggled with the most recent passing of a friend, and was finding support through both an in person social community and their social media community, but was feeling extremely lonely in their grief and loss. The Social Bloom can really expand on what might be going on with your broader network in relationship to grief and loss. For instance, how have you been relating to social media prior to the loss? And now, how are you relating? What has been helpful about any shifts and what has not been helpful with your social media? Similarly, how is that going with your in-person network? Typically, our network of people are those rooting for us, and yet in grief and loss, it can feel like many of them are not because they do not know how to respond and have complex lives they are living. And so it can feel very isolating, hence the loneliness in this social realm.

Consider how you might engage with the Social Bloom to improve your livelihood, and that includes potentially letting somebody in your social network know how you are feeling with your grief and loss and how others can support you. You may realize that there are some people in your social network you really want to get to know better and have not had the opportunity, and recognize this is a suitable time in your life to get to know those people better. So, you reach out. On the other end of it, there may be people in your social circle who are responding negatively to your grief, thinking you might need to get over it quickly or judging your grief response. And that is not helpful. Having to deal with those hard conversations amidst the grief is really challenging. Talk about some strategies for how to deal with hard conversations with a friend or professional, and part of that work includes being clear and setting boundaries. Direct and effective communication in grief and loss is HARD. A lot of what is happening in the social space relates to personal work and interpersonal work that is going on as you navigate your new world. So, it is heavy. It takes a lot of time, practice, and energy. Give yourself a break if you feel a conversation did not go well. Give the other person a bit of grace too. Root into your abilities to communicate in a way that works for you.

Getting support from others on social media may be helpful for some and not as helpful for others. It is okay to make changes to what you are doing on social media if it helps you to do so. People in your social network, which includes relationships outside of close family and close friends, may want to support you. Let them know what is helpful and what is not.

- What social practices have been helpful to you during your grieving process?

- How does your social media support and/or hinder your grief?

- What is coming up for you with your relationship to your social network?

- What do you want and need from your social network?

Sociological Bloom

"I am frustrated. I entered perimenopause, and I am grieving that no one has normalized talking about this and the symptoms that accompany this stage of life. These are much more complex than a simple fix, and no one is talking about supporting women during this phase like they do in other phases of people's lives. This phase is hard. I am more tired. My hair is different. So is my skin. I am gaining weight, even though I exercise. I grieve that society does not talk about this phase of life more outwardly, and I grieve that women are not supported more." This individual tried navigating various health care systems, approaches, and modalities to find strategies that work for her as she noticed a substantial shift in her wellbeing as she entered perimenopause. There is a lot to grieve, from the lack of society's awareness of and support for this stage of life to various lifestyle changes. I have heard similar sentiments from others in this phase of life too.

Sometimes sociological conditions block our abilities to heal how we need to heal and to receive support how we need to receive support. We can focus on finding support with friends and possibly support groups while accessing various healing modalities. Those supporting a griever can help to build awareness about topics (such as perimenopause) by sharing stories and advocating for better support, for example.

"I am so mad at the people looking out for my loved one. How did they not catch this before it was too late?" I have heard this multiple times. These are painful sentiments that add a lot of heartache in the grieving process while opening us up to learning more about ourselves and the world. They also need to be explored for healing. Sometimes people want to explore the medical system to find a way to advocate for better care, more research, or more funding, and other times, people want to write a complex letter to the system that they send or tear up and throw away as part of their healing. Systems can fail us in our grief. Systems break down constantly; it is the promise of the ever-changing, dynamic, and chaotic world we live in, and yet, we can channel our grief to work toward more promising changes. This is not something that one has to do right away or take on finding a cure for something. They can be small, subtle, beautiful changes that you tend to as you engage your life wholeheartedly. What is your grief telling you about the systems you have encountered and how you can be a force for hope?

Answer the following questions from a space of curiosity and less judgment. You have the right to interrogate these systems and how they are impacting you and your grief. Focus on what you can do to support your health and grieving needs.

- Which of these systems: medical, education, and/or health-care have influenced you the most in your grief?

- What helps you navigate these systems in your grief?

- How does your local culture respond to grief and loss?

- How does your education and professional training inform your grief?

Chapter 8 Exercise

Choose one of the Blooms from this chapter. Is this a Bloom you noted from the Chapter Six exercise? Journal or reflect on the questions asked about that Bloom in this chapter. Are there any other questions that come up related to that Bloom? In reflecting on that Bloom, does it lead you to reflect on any other Blooms?

Select the Bloom, either internal or external, you want to explore the most. Is it the one you felt most ambiguous about from the Chapter Six exercise or has that shifted for you?

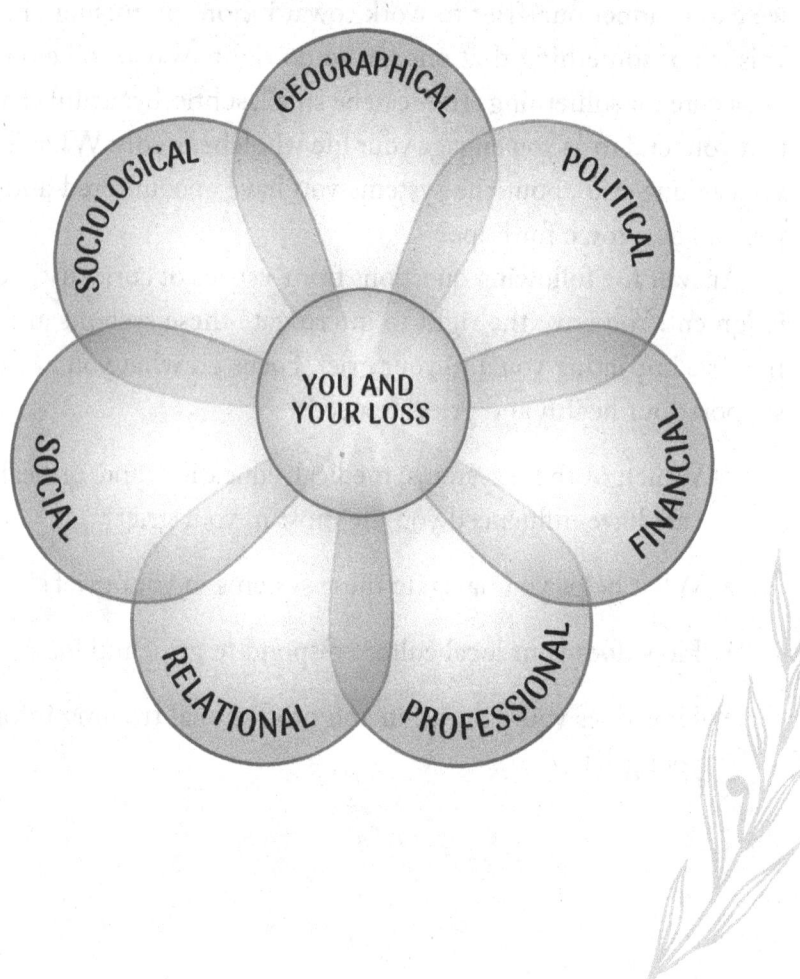

The Path

The path,
navigated with strengths and entered through the paradox,
To new potential, new experiences, new living.

Juxtaposing pathways brings clarity,
Opening oneself up whole-heartedly to possibilities,
Bringing in the hope of tomorrow and cradling the sadness of the past.

The path,
treaded with determination, taken with small steps,
To new potential, new experiences, new living.

Surrendering to the complexity, losing clarity,
Engaging with curiosity, gaining understanding,
Basking in the hope of today and tending to feelings of yesterday.

The path,
approached with ease and hardship, walked with mistakes and honesty,
To new potential, new experiences, new living.

Chapter 9

Opening Yourself to the BloomPath®

*"Take the first step in faith. You don't have to see
the whole staircase, just take the first step."*

—Often attributed to Martin Luther King Jr., unknown

For the opening of the Blooms of your grief, you reflect on your wants
and needs regarding your grief and losses. You listen whole-heartedly
to who you are becoming. Often, grief forces you to interrogate your
wants and needs. What draws you into your more authentic self? As
part of the opening of your Blooms, you acknowledge and discover the
areas of strength and difficulty in your grief and loss. Take a moment
to reflect on your strengths; something positive someone noticed in
you that you did not notice in yourself prior to your grief. Everyone
has innate strengths, and part of opening your Blooms here is recognizing your strengths, bringing you closer to your own authenticity.
Some people relate to their strengths such as their values or personality traits that make them thrive in addition to things they are good at.

Building on your reflection about your ambiguity in grief and
exploring the questions for each Bloom, there are additional ways
to engage with the BloomPath®, such as a reflection tool or as a
compass to help you make a change that you want to make. And
there is a structured way to use it for deliberate hopeful intentions

and well-defined plans to meet your goals discussed throughout the following chapters. While this book takes you through that process, please note that many of the clients I work with use the BloomPath® in their own unique ways.

Sometimes we start growing out of some of the most challenging moments in our lives. My first experience with this happened before I was born. The doctors could not find my heartbeat part way through the pregnancy. They had to complete an in-utero exploration to find my heartbeat. Eventually, I was born, and my heart was fine except for a minor murmur. I started as a broken seed, and I cultivated that seed with hopes and dreams, determination and sensitivity, and achievement and judgment until the death of my daughter. Then, I learned to let life cultivate me. Nicknamed "Sprocket" from an early age, I was a high-energy kid with a lot of scholastic determination and a sensitivity toward what was being felt in a room, aside from what was being said. The sensitivity that was so encompassing necessitated purposeful cultivation that I would not start tending to until my thirties.

Just as my daughter's death had opened me up to a more compassionate life, my determination helped me grapple with my ambiguity to a new way of being and living. That opening also helped me make small shifts in my daily life and understanding who I really am when I make decisions from a place of love. While I continue to try to lead life in various ways, I am much more open to life leading me to fulfill dreams and ambitions much larger than I ever expected. By opening to the paradox of letting life lead me, I have less ambiguity and more clarity about my connectedness to the world and the life that I am meant to live. I now find purpose through my strengths and help others recognize theirs too.

In grief, it can be challenging to notice your strengths for two reasons: you are changing, so your strengths may be shifting; and the complexity of feelings we hold as a griever can make it difficult to access positive emotional mindsets that remind us of our own strengths. Sometimes having conversations with others about your strengths may serve as a gentle reminder of who you are and what you are capable of. When we consider strengths, we are also open to being stuck or creating movement or doing both with them. This helps us be available to our needs while participating in our own opening up and forgoing panicking when we are stuck. This allows us to embrace curiosity and patience from a strengths-based perspective.

In addition to your strengths, consider grief expert Thomas Attig's process of relearning the world[13]. Attig includes various areas that one relearns through grief and loss. Three include relearning: physical surroundings, relationships, and one's self (Attig 1996, p. 109-116).

The physical surroundings may be an empty room of someone who died, or a half of a bed after a divorce, and in my own personal journey with my car accident, having to relearn how to navigate my home with one hand for a few months. The physical surroundings mostly relate to the Geographical Bloom. What are examples from your own life where you have needed to relearn your physical surroundings?

Second is relearning relationships. For example, how has your relationship changed with those around you? For some, they may be relearning their relationships after the ambiguous loss of an estranged family member[14]. For others, they may be navigating new relationships with those who have entered their lives as a direct result of a loss experience, or someone may be learning to parent as a single parent or wondering how to parent a child who died. Relearning relationships relates to the Relational and Social Blooms.

The third aspect of Attig's work deals with relearning your identity. Questions such as, "Who am I since this loss?" or "What are my values now?" or even more acutely, "How do I get through this day when my prior coping skills are not working for me now?" As part of the opening of your roots, you are aware about what you are relearning. These are additional questions to consider when you think about your strengths. These aspects relate to the Identity Bloom.

When we are open to entering the paradox of our life, we create buoyancy, resiliency, and more open heartedness in our lives. Grief is challenging, yet it opens us up to new ways of thinking. The paradox is something that I started to understand after the death of my daughter because I was certainly trying to control life instead of leaning into it, which meant that I was judging unkindly and thinking that my life was going to work out how I planned. I have since been engaging with the concept of the paradox. Part of it cannot be explained. It is a window into knowing that there is so much more than what we see. Prior to Evelyn's death, I was making decisions based out of fear and based out of a deep want to be wanted in life. But it was not until I entered that paradox that I could meet those roots and needs of mine and explore old ways of thinking and begin to unwind into new ways of viewing myself, others, and the world.

The paradox is holding space for multiple theories, ideas, creativity, pain, joy, and not knowing to embark on more mindful decision making from an open heart and open mind, actively choosing from a place of love. Prior to the death of my daughter, I was not aware of this space nor was I even open to being in this space. What helped me enter this space was the fact that the circle of life philosophy was upended when my daughter died before me. I was forced to enter and relearn my world and make meaning from my world. The BloomPath® helps you enter a space of paradox too.

The paradox is also all the confusion that cannot be explained. The paradox disrupts old ideas and more importantly old ways of being to become someone a little bit different. The paradox allows us to open to mystery and access our inner wisdom. The paradox is a bunch of in between and a curious understanding of similarities and differences, opening us up to both discontent and gratitude. It causes us to interrogate our logic and feel into our deeper understandings of ourselves and the world. When I find myself existing in the paradox, I become more of myself which, in itself, is a paradox. By understanding that I am connected to the world around me and the people around me but also root into who I am, I recognize the paradox. I acknowledge the mystery of the human experience and embrace the known and unknown. So, at the simplest level the paradox is the "both and." I am both saddened by the loss of Evelyn, and I am grateful that this loss has opened me up to new ways of thinking and living. What is your both and?

This paradox shows up in grief because most types of losses upend our world and cause us to relate to ourselves and to others in different and unexpected ways. There is so much more than what we understand, and there is so much more than what we feel and think. By engaging in the paradox, we can hold on to things more lightly and more tenderly. We can be more compassionate versions of ourselves. We can be okay with not knowing and still be curious. We can be our authentic selves, and we can be wholehearted. The paradox includes bringing yourself the world's most inner wisdom to connect with at a level that is freeing and that brings a new type of life into our lives. This is all possible in our grief. It may not be at the beginning of a grief experience as you are maybe initially feeling some numbness or shock, but it could be many months or years later. People engage with their grief differently and on different timelines, and the paradox allows for that.

When you are open to reflecting on the nuances within each of the thirteen Blooms and with the BloomPath® as a whole, you can make decisions out of a place of love, strength, meaningful information, and authenticity.

One of the recurring themes I hear from many individuals is about finding new pathways forward to hold both ends of a spectrum. Living here and hoping for what was or will be, feeling both fear and love, sadness, and hope. Grief is one of the few spaces that opens us up to that paradox, and when we enter the paradox to disrupt old thinking patterns that are not kind to ourselves and others, we find our inner light that brings our authentic selves into the world. It may be hard and comforting to hold the complexity of grief. One client said they felt sad about their friend's death and that sadness led them to a newfound love for life.

Chapter 9 Exercise

What are your strengths? How are they shifting? How do you want to use them to tend to your grief and the Bloom(s) you explore?

How do you feel about the paradox of grief?

What are some positive moments that you have had because of your grief? How are you letting life lead you? How does this relate to the loss you are exploring with the BloomPath®?

Chapter 10

Tending Blooms

"It's the little things that always tend to grow."

—John Coggins

Now that you have reflected on your strengths and the paradox of your situation, try tending to your Blooms. You get to highlight areas in your life where you are stuck and where there is movement for you, which helps you prioritize what you want to be more aware of, be more resolute about, both within your external and internal life. Sometimes tending is merely observing and other times it is pruning away things that are not working for you. Other times it is growing new seeds and utilizing new strategies. Keep in mind, when things are hard or you are not seeing progress quickly, it may feel that they are not working for you. That is part of the complexity of human growth. So, sometimes it makes sense to continue with what you are doing before trying something else. Other times, it can simply mean a small adjustment in your life, to continue tending to what you need to within yourself.

You can also clear or tend to emotional clutter. What thoughts and emotions are causing you the most suffering? How can you utilize resources to help you with those? As we tend to our grief and losses, we often notice the need to clear emotional clutter in our lives to be able to tend to other areas of our lives more fully. This can mean reflections, journaling, counseling, coaching, movement, or more modalities for exploration. Clearing emotional clutter is about bringing awareness to what you are feeling and digging deep into the nuance of these feelings, so you can understand your emotional life. As you tend to your Blooms, you will see how those emotions impact behavior, thoughts, and overall wellness. The rawness of these feelings in grief may require several types of tending to at various points in your grief. That looks different throughout your lifespan of holding grief. For example, an individual explained how they were not grieving their parent how they thought they needed and wanted and decided to focus on the Emotional Bloom as part of their healing.

To help you embrace your emotions and care for yourself, follow these steps:

1. Feel your emotions by noticing your thoughts, behaviors, and internal changes such as heart rate.

2. Create nuance about your feelings by framing them with as many words to describe them as you can. What words come up for you?

3. Tend to the feelings with an array of strategies based on the words that have the most impact related to your feelings. You can do this by simply observing them and being curious about them without judgment.

4. There are so many more words for our grief feelings than currently exist in English. For example, if I am feeling sad, what are synonyms for this word? Maybe I am upset, frustrated, lonely, and more. When I notice more words to describe this feeling, I can then tend to those feelings. It is a lot easier for me to know what I am upset, frustrated, lonely, and sad about than simply only recognizing that I am sad. Naming and describing emotions helps us heal. From there you can tend to your emotions by applying strategies to address your feelings. Maybe you will talk

with someone about them. Maybe you will go on a walk. Maybe you listen to music. Maybe you create something. These are examples of tending to your emotions, and you have many more options to use that are not discussed in this book, but that authors, counselors, and experts have shared. See the Feelings Exploration Example for a summary of how the Feelings Exploration Activity may be used in practice.

Feelings Exploration Example

Steps
- *feel your feelings and note the feeling word that sticks out to you the most;*
- *gain more words and understanding for that feeling; and*
- *tend to the feeling word(s) you are most impacted by in the moment.*

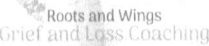
Roots and Wings
Grief and Loss Coaching

Example of how to use the steps
- Word: *Sad*
- Describe word: melancholy, depressed, tired
- Synonyms, phrases, metaphors that describe the word: candle blown out in my life, angry that I'm sad
- Where this word shows up in my life lately: can't be sad when I need to be
- How I respond: turn sadness inward on myself to self hatred, anger, and depression; close off, rest, nap
- How would I respond to someone else with this feeling: Text them; stop by their place; let them know that whatever they are feeling is okay and normal; and/or give a hug if they are huggers, for example
- These responses would work for me with adjustments, and I will try giving myself a "hug" by noticing that I am feeling depressed right now, and I will try gentle movement, such as walking, to tend to this feeling.

After you have opened your Blooms with your strengths and are embracing the paradox, then tended to those Blooms, your next step in the following chapters is to cultivate one or a few Blooms to open yourself to the possibility for growth. For example, are you wanting to change something geographically, which could mean anything from changing the layout of your bedroom to moving across the world? Or do you want to explore your spirituality more intentionally? Maybe you want to change your career or go back to your prior career with newfound clarity. In the grow phase, it is possible to set newfound or prior unexplored goals with a purposeful and hopeful method. In the following chapters, you will have the opportunity to work through hopeful exercises that are thoughtful and strategic to fit you and your circumstances.

Revisiting the example of Lani, she realized she needed time to listen to herself and what her wants and needs were telling her. Her relationship was starting to grow with her new friend from the support group, and this was an invaluable outlet for her as she leaned into being supported by a friend and being a friend too. The reciprocity of their relationship was met with ease and comfort. As she started to Bloom into a new chapter of her life, she began to understand she had other wants and needs too. Her wants and needs were supported by her spouse, and she wanted to better understand herself. She focused on the Relational Bloom and the Identity Bloom. She and her husband continued marital counseling, and she leaned into better understanding herself outside of her caretaker role. She began to engage in both old and new hobbies and carved out time for listening to music. She started to feel a little lighter and opened herself up to being okay with the paradox and sitting with her contrasting feelings and the gray area she was now opening herself up to exploring.

For now, create space to complete the exercise at the end of this chapter. When is the last time that you had the opportunity to sit with your wants and needs and let whatever is opening naturally get the tending to that it needs to make it grow? We do not get those opportunities often, and yet, they can be so empowering. Maybe take some time to talk with a friend about your own paradox and how that may relate to the Blooms in this book. Sit open hearted and open minded. Focus on your breath and call in to your life the beginning of this process for you. If you are currently early in your grieving, it may make sense to be in the numbness of it all, and that is okay too. When the time feels right, or at least almost right, engage in your paradox by opening and tending. Maybe you want to explore more writings or maybe you want to listen to music. Perhaps you want to engage with friends and/or family, or you prefer to journal alone. Listen to yourself and what you are open to trying. Hold yourself gently throughout the entire process, just as you would a Bloom.

Chapter 10 Exercise

- What are you noticing about the Bloom(s) you are exploring? What is naturally opening to you the most through the Bloom? What about the least in that Bloom?

- What needs the most tending to from your Bloom(s)?

- What are the little things that are starting to grow with hope?

- Carry your reflection into Chapter 11 to begin opening the Bloom(s) that you want to heal. As you explore the Bloom(s), be open to shifting your exploration to another Bloom or add additional Blooms to focus.

Chapter 11

Growing with Intention

*"Hope is holding a creative tension between what is and
what could and should be, each day doing something
to narrow the distance between the two."*

—Parker Palmer

In this chapter, you will take a moment to consider which Bloom
opens for you naturally in your grief now and use that Bloom as an
anchor to set intentions for yourself, guided by C.R. Snyder's Hope
Theory[15].

Sometimes goals can help us re-orient to ourselves and the environment around us when experiencing grief. Goals can support us to
get out of the house again or to take a walk. On the other hand, when
focused on the goal alone, we lose sight of the stirring and the beauty
of what is happening within us to create meaningful change for ourselves amidst the pain and heartache of loss. A dear friend told me
about goal-directed behavior, "There is a time to swim and a time to
float on your back. When you float on your back, you take the time to
stop swimming, and still, end up somewhere else. You leave the door
open. When aimed at a particular goal, you may lose sight of what
shows up in your space. When floating on your back, you unknowingly create movement, and you made the intention to float on your
back." Interweaving this type of goal-directed behavior with more
purposeful direction may be a balanced way to approach goal setting.

This is why I appreciate C.R. Snyder's Hope Theory. His work is situated in the field of positive psychology, and it focuses on finding your agency and pathways. C.R. Snyder offers the following definition of Hope Theory: "Hope is a positive motivational state that is based on an interactively derived sense of successful (a) agency (goal-directed energy), and (b) pathways (planning to meet goals)."[16] As part of the theory, focus is shifted to agency and pathways. Agency includes assumptions about who you are and what you can learn. As your assumptions and beliefs about who you are and what you can learn are shifting in grief and loss, take time to reflect about who you are and what you can learn to process your grief and your desires for your new life. This is a helpful theory as we must now take a different pathway and approach than we previously had envisioned for ourselves.

You can use Hope Theory to set goals while staying true to yourself. Pathways are your steps to reach a goal, and they are situated within time, starting with your first tiny step and mapping out your additional steps until you have identified a pathway that may work for you to reach your desired state of being, action-oriented goal, or steps to a new or next pathway. You are more likely to actualize your pathways when you have clear steps that are not only manageable but nearly so attainable they are but a microscopic shift in your current way of being and/or acting, a blend of floating and trying.

Pay attention to what you can do rather than what you cannot do so that you create the neural pathways in your brain to focus on the hope-directed goal you may have. When you focus on what you can, you create hope for yourself. In the earliest parts of grief, it may be about getting out of bed to sit in a chair. As time moves on, you move into a new life and may want to direct your energy to what you *can* do to draw you into your authenticity and hope.

Jane, a fifty-year-old woman, was grieving when her husband lost his longtime job and was no longer able to work due to various life factors. She had not been in the paid workforce for fifteen years, and as part of their new life circumstances, she was considering going back to full-time employment. As part of understanding her wants and desires, she first considered her agency by asking questions such as, "Who am I? What do I want my days to look like? What skills do I have? What am I willing to learn? Who can help me with these questions? What activities can I engage in to gain more clarity, such as creative acts, career assessments, etc.? What am I grieving about the loss of my husband's work?"

After contemplating possible moves, Jane decided she wanted to work toward getting a job at the local bookstore or at a local engineering firm. She first created this step: meet with individuals at each of these locations to learn more about the work options available in the local community. She scaffolded that back to a manageable first step: write down five informational interview questions for each agency, and call each individual in the appropriate department tomorrow to set up a time to meet.

Understanding your agency using small steps may help create pathways that are more easily followed, more motivating to start, and more fulfilling. Focusing on agency may take weeks, months, and even longer. These timelines are highly personal. As you gain more self-awareness, work to create a step-by-step guide for yourself to take micro-steps to move closer to your wants and needs.

Scott was grieving the death of his wife of two years. They were both teachers. Scott took bereavement leave for a month then started back at work, not feeling like himself. He was unclear if it was grief or the discontent for various aspects of his life. He worked to develop his agency, continuing to actively grieve his wife. He spent time after school in therapy, journaling, exercising, crying, resting, and more. This continued for many months. While his grief may have felt a bit lighter, he was still unsure about who he was in the world after this devastating loss. He took time to sit with his mind, heart, and emotions to clarify his direction in life.

Here is what he started to uncover about his agency: he liked his work and his community. He knew he wanted to explore more about himself, so rather than a week-long trip, he took a summer-long job across the country. He journaled about his summer and talked to many people. He realized this pathway was somewhat helpful for him to better understand himself and his grief, so he constructed a different pathway based on his new self-understanding. The following school year, as part of the BloomPath®, he decided to focus on his physical health. He started with a small step of running one lap at the school track before going home. He saw a therapist and worked toward more self-understanding. As part of constructing Scott's pathway, he had to explore more about himself and improve his physical health.

Both stories about Jane and Scott are vastly different, and that is one of the key points about understanding Hope Theory. You have your agency that no one else has—you know what motivates you, how you are changing, and more, and that is why discovering more about your agency and pathways can lead you to more fulfilling goals. Your strengths are part of your agency along with your understanding of what motivates you and how you are changing as you grieve. Do you always have to be so resolute? Not necessarily. It is okay to be stuck or to stand still and just wait, at least a moment so you do not force something that does not need to happen. Embrace the unknown, uncovering what your grief is showing you each day.

In the growth stage of the model, you are going to set small pathways to open yourself up to intentional growth within one or multiple Blooms. Find a moment to grow a small action-oriented step out of that moment. Maybe that includes something like continuing reflection or continuing journaling. Maybe it includes making a phone call to an individual or to a provider or to a close friend. Maybe it is going on an extra walk each week than what you currently are doing. The whole point about growing is that we grow by very, very small action steps that we deliberately put into place. These are not big substantial changes that happen overnight or within a few days.

James Clear explains habit formation and how you can make something a habit by starting very small, tying it to something that you are already doing in your day, and reinforcing that with something positive[17]. One other piece here is acknowledging that there is another layer of self-love in this process, and that is taking ownership of all the stumbles that will happen and facing shame and taking ownership of your growth. This is hard, and you can do hard things. Sometimes the shame and missteps may feel overwhelming; remember, your brain is reorienting to the world as you grieve, so be gentle on yourself for the mistakes you make and tend to your feelings of shame or guilt with compassion and understanding.

As you gain new insights from agency and pathways, it may be worth exploring goals more in relationship to grief and loss. Goals can range from lofty, such as integrating coaching concepts in the way you learn, work, and live, or to relocate or go back to school, to simple, such as completely cleaning the office desktop or making a necessary phone call. And the consideration of goals, through agency, pathways, and the value of the outcome, can happen over the course of decades or be as swift as the blink of an eye.

There are three stages to setting goals in Hope Theory. The first stage is pre-event, the decision-making process of what goals to consider and the value of the possible outcomes. This stage includes the learning, assumptions, and experiences of the past mixed with hopes, dreams, and fears of the future. The next stage is during the action steps themselves, when immersed in the process. During this stage, action is measured with results and leads to either staying engaged, and even continuing to increase engagement, to choosing to take a break, or stopping and deciding to disengage. The final stage is reflection and learning, and absorption of experiences that happens when the results tumble in. This final stage feeds back into ideas and assumptions about agency and possible paths, completing the cycle and starting a new cycle anew. Obstacles are also a key part of Hope Theory. They are necessary for optimal performance and learning.

Using these steps of Hope Theory helps you identify small goals and foreseeable barriers to those and opportunities for those so you can produce a clear action plan and have clarity about how you create movement toward your goal. The BloomPath® helps people gain more clarity in a very confusing time in their lives. Also, I recognize the need for adventure and the need for freedom, for lack of better words, to live a life and just kind of go with the flow, and this type of goal setting still allows you to do that but just gives you a little bit of that space to be more intentional with how you do that, how you go with the flow, how you want to live your life, and who you want to be and how you want to grieve.

This is what is so hopeful about Hope Theory. You have the agency to construct different pathways if they are not working for you and adjust your goals if they are not working for you. You can move onto plans b, c, and/or d if needed. Grief often reveals how little control we have, so Hope Theory gives you an anchor to create movement for your wants and needs. It also helps you explore back-up options that you now may need to consider.

When Lani completed the exercise at the end of this chapter, here's what she came up with:

Vision for self: I want to better know who I am, Identity Bloom.

Short term goal: I will try one new experience each week starting next week for six weeks.

Resources needed to achieve short term goal: Time, intention, money. I will budget up to $30 for each new experience, some will not cost additional money, and some will.

Roadblocks and opportunities for short term goal: motivation, tiredness, busy schedule, opportunity—say no to something I am doing that isn't a good fit and try something else; shift one experience I am having every week to make it more suitable for my needs; try reading a new genre or listening to a new podcast.

Additional thoughts, feelings, intuitions about vision and goal: I am tired. I have just recently returned to work after using bereavement leave after the death of my dad. I just want to rest. However, I am feeling some motivation to try something different that is healthy for me and that brings me into the person I am becoming, and I want to do something new while also finding time and space to rest. I want to try something by myself, and in the future, add in my partner and friends.

My first next step: Commit to going to a local music event by putting it in my calendar.

My second next step: Buy tickets for the event.

My third next step: Be open to the spectrum of feelings I have before, during, and after the concert.

Vision for self: No matter whether the event is a bust or amazing, I will feel good about myself for trying something new, and I will learn something new about myself.

Even though the event opened her up to more feelings of sadness, it also expanded her capacity to feel joy for the first time in a long time. Lani realized how much she missed live music, and she decided she would make concert going a part of her life more often.

Chapter 11 Exercise

Apply the exercise to the loss you are exploring with the BloomPath® and the Bloom(s) you are exploring.

Hopeful Exercise

Short term goal (very small, a small stretch, action oriented, and timebound):

Resources needed to achieve short term goal:

Roadblocks and opportunities for short term goal:

Additional thoughts, feelings, intuitions about vision and goal:

My first next step:

My second next step:

My third next step:

Vision for Self:

Chapter 12

Flourishing with Authenticity

During our grief, we can feel highly vulnerable, and it can be especially difficult to let others see us in our moments of despair, our moments of depression, and even in moments of finding ourselves. In a coaching practice session, I asked another coach what it's like to be seen. And that was a moment that I felt my own soul breaking open to better understand what it really means to be seen in this world. I remember she struggled with the question, especially in that instant and eventually mentioned to some degree how hard it is to be seen. In our ordinary moments, it can feel too vulnerable to be seen, so when we layer in moments where we are actively grieving, it can feel impossible to let others in or to let others see you.

Recently, I went on a run and took a completely different route than I typically do and ran along one of the main thoroughfares in town, and despite very heavy traffic, I was not necessarily concerned of being hit by a vehicle, but I was scared of being seen.

I had to check in with myself and understand why running among many vehicles where people could see me run felt so vulnerable for me. I am not the fastest or most graceful runner, and I am certainly not the most in shape, so I was scared that I might be seen in a not-so-perfect condition even though I love running. I come up with my best ideas when I am running, as movement has been so helpful in my grief and in both my professional and personal lives. So being seen as a runner is like being broken open in a raw vulnerable way. This brokenness exposes the layers of the self, which is fractured, imperfect. And when others see that in us, it's scary and we want to be able to have some shield so that we don't have to feel the difficult emotions and can live in a way that keeps us hidden. In fact, when I am running, I do not need a shield. I certainly could use water, but I had to check in with myself in this instance to say it is okay to be seen like this, seen far from perfect, running.

What makes being seen in grief and loss so challenging is that most people do not know how to respond to grievers in a way that lets them be themselves while also providing hope. For those family and friends, walking alongside the griever can be very frustrating because in our society we want pinpoint answers when there are not any. We want to be able to say to our friend or family member, "It'll be okay," or "You should get some help." What we can do instead is sit with the griever and listen to what it is they genuinely want and need and how that can be provided. Remove your own agenda, and listen to the individual, then reflect back what you are hearing and ask if they would be open to continuing these conversations with you consistently. Sometimes you are not the person to have these conversations with and other times you may be. If you are the one grieving, ask your family or friends to do this for you.

Being seen running is different from being seen in our despair and grief. So, think about that exposure. That rawness, being peeled back or completely shattered, and that opening in grief that happens as we experience loss. That does not necessarily go away, but you now see the world and yourself in a different way. You can be okay with those wounds. That hole. That shattering. And build yourself a new life and new hope to wear that hole and let in the light. And to wear that hole becomes so that you can be seen authentically as your true selves. Someone once mentioned to me that it is interesting that hole is spelled h-o-l-e or another spelling of whole, another meaning of hole, is w-h-o-l-e. Hole lives inside whole. To be whole, you need to break. You need a hole to be broken to open up to new possibilities. We are beings now broken open to possibilities in our grief.

Being seen is blooming into your authenticity.

As you discover ways to meet your short-term goal from Chapter 11, it may be helpful to consider how you are blooming into your new self with both authenticity and purpose.

Authenticity

Some Blooms open naturally. Before loss, one may relate to life differently than after loss. That was the case for me in many ways, and at the root of the difference was my spiritual shift, which broadened me to my authenticity and understanding of the paradox. Prior to the death of my daughter, the world held color yet included significant space for black and white—black and white thinking, black and white understanding of the basics of color, and so much more. But, after loss, everything awakened to colors, colors I had never seen before, vibrant, and yet dull, with new thoughts, feelings, and emotions, much more colorful than ever before and eventually much kinder.

Spirituality has always been a part of my life. I relied on my Catholic faith to get me through various points in my childhood, adolescence, and young adulthood. In college, however, I became frustrated with the inability to access God's love and to access my authenticity, which I now define as my goodness in my strengths and compassionate understandings from my challenges. After the death of my daughter, I experienced many spiritual moments that brought me comfort and mysticism. That brought me curiosity. That brought me faith and doubt, frustration and contentment. These are all emotions, thoughts, and moments that I have grappled with in my grief. In my healing, I noticed the parallel between what spirituality can do and what God or an external force knows about grief and how that is lived out in your own grief. Whether you believe in God, nature, the connectedness of things, or the seasons of life—whatever it is in relationship to something greater than yourself, the Spiritual Bloom provides the space for you to explore that nuance that exists in the in-between spaces and may co-exist with the paradox. For me, the Spiritual Bloom opened, and I needed to find ways to access that opening. I surrendered to my journey, and I realized that I could start working toward a more robust understanding of my spirituality through my agency and pathways.

Since the death of Evelyn, I have had truly mystical experiences. As part of hope and setting goals, I started to open myself up to leaning into these spiritual puzzles. The Halloween after her death, a few months after she died, I was struggling. I was going to drive to my sister's house to spend the holiday there, but the moment I got in the car, I could only drive thirty minutes until I just broke down and turned right around, pulling over on the side of the road feeling both numb and anxious as I called her to let her know I would not make it. Tears barely streaming down my face, I drove back to my home, and I spent the evening with my neighbors, handing out candy to trick or treaters. I was sad and grieving my daughter and my inability to drive over thirty minutes away. After I went to bed around midnight, the front door opened, and I ran downstairs and could not find anything but the door open, so I went back to bed and next to me on my bed was a nonbinary red-headed angel telling me that they were there to take my pain away. I felt and saw this divine being at a level I could not have anticipated and still cannot describe. I know our minds can do strange things to open the window to a world that is so much more than what we understand.

Another experience that has been recurring for the past five years is that my daughter Evelyn is in a field of the most full and beautiful yet light and airy wildflowers, and we meet there. When this vision comes to me, she is always meeting me at the age she would be and not as an infant. It is incredible and nothing I created to deal with my grief. It just shows up. Grief shows up in a mystical way and we cannot ascertain that there is any specific pattern for it because it is something that is beyond what a surgeon can take a slice out of and then send to a lab to be examined. Grief is hard, possibly mystical, beautiful, and meaningful. Grief opens us up to our authenticity and may be a source for personal development. I have learned that we should talk more about grief, be open to experiences we have not encountered before, that may be deeply personal and yet collectively felt, somewhat understood, and shared in meaningful ways.

As part of my goal-directed behavior, I opened myself to these new spiritual experiences to bring them into my life for new meaning and hope, which helped me root into my personality strengths of positivity and curiosity, growing my authenticity. This is much clearer now than it was to me then because I was not working from any map or framework at the time.

While the Spiritual Bloom was a key focus in the latitude of my grief, other Blooms may start to naturally open in grief for you. Different Blooms may open more naturally than others with each of your grief occurrences, and it may be that with each of your grief experiences, a different Bloom may draw you in more than another one. You may also notice a sprout within one of the Blooms that is not opening naturally but you are drawn to it. That is where scaffolding your understanding of yourself in the context of that Bloom is significant and may take more intentional work to move from a sprout to a Bloom and live authentically.

What does it mean to live an authentic life in relationship to grief and loss? Grief may serve as an amplifier to understanding your emotions, to making shifts in relationships, to rooting into old habits and discovering new ones. When grieving, you can either break down walls and become more authentic or put up more walls and hide who you really are. This is not a finite process, and one may waiver between authenticity and hiding before Blooming into who they are becoming. I have been reflecting on this paradox since the death of my daughter. Prior to that, I had many questions about philosophies and my own familial systems and roots. But these thoughts and feelings were expressed based on thinking and judgment. It was all based in "pull yourself up by your bootstraps" mindset, with little regard for compassion, failure, or mistakes. This type of thinking is not helpful in grief and loss.

Various people would tell me, just three months after my loss, that I needed to get it together and move on. These orders from others were not helpful and made my loss more painful. I have since noticed how much this type of thinking and feeling permeates our culture and how toxic it may be, especially in grief and loss. People want to shut off their uncomfortable emotions and want you to do the same and cope with them in ways that were learned behaviors and not necessarily effective. We are emotional beings just as much as we are thinking beings, and we need the space to honor what is happening internally in our grief. There are no quick fixes, and going through grief takes time and, often, kind support.

From my grief, the type of authenticity that I am now more open to is a bit softer, a bit kinder, and a bit freer. Authenticity is not about checking the boxes for success, and it is not about living a life that someone else has envisioned for you or societal expectations. Yet all these things matter, and they all swim in the background of living out our authenticity.

Our authenticity includes what our heart, mind, and soul know to be true for ourselves. What is good and kind for others and oneself. What is empowering, supports your growth, to become wiser, and to embrace hard emotions. This authenticity is lived out determinedly, and it is lived out by being you. You were made to shine as your authentic self, and you are here with specific gifts, talents, mindsets, loves, hobbies, relationships, and more to give to the world, so that you live as your authentic self and support others to do so as well. Understanding that what is permeating the background, societal norms, and structured workdays, for example, does not impact your ability to live and thrive as the complex human that you are. We are sensitive beings, and we are meant to engage with our sensitive side just as much as the logical. How is authenticity showing up in each of your Blooms? Where are you feeling your most genuine? Where are you stuck?

As you root into your authenticity and engage with your grief, uncertainty may reveal itself. For some, trying to find their way through their feelings in these moments can be challenging. Sometimes it is easier to only use our minds to move forward, and we know as humans that is not possible. We are complicated beings that need nuanced and holistic support through grief and loss. When I was grieving in the early months after the death of my daughter, I met with my former professor on a college campus, and he said, "Eryn, you cannot think your way out of this." These words have stuck with me for over ten years, and at the time, they sounded so strange. I did not think I was thinking my way through this. I feel like I tend to be an emotional being, and yet, when I reflected on those words, I realized I was putting up a shield to access all the range of emotions that I needed to access to heal.

When fear takes hold of your grief, you cannot grieve as yourself and may hold on so tightly that it hurts. What happens when you root into who you are rather than holding false identities, false expectations, and holding on too tightly? These questions consistently show up in grief and loss. One individual I spoke with said that they had been holding onto the identity of caretaker for so long that they did not know how to be anyone or do anything differently. And yet, they wanted to make shifts. They considered how they wanted to integrate their caretaking abilities into this next chapter of their life and what they wanted to let go of and what they wanted to carry forward.

When considering how you embark on your journey, surrender to your authenticity. First, open to what is broken, imperfect in yourself, and what you regard as your strengths, talents, or something about yourself that lets the light in. Imagine yourself at peace with your imperfections. What is something you find contentment about yourself? Consider your inner peace—what is that? Where is authenticity showing up in each of your Blooms? Which Blooms are you stuck in your authenticity? Now, create moments to explore that authenticity. Take two separate times throughout the day and spend one minute checking in with yourself. Ask yourself, "How can I open myself to my authenticity over the next ten minutes of my day?" Keep doing this consistently over the course of a week, a month, or more.

Chapter 12 Exercise

We need safe spaces to be our authentic selves to explore our losses with the BloomPath®.

Visit a space/location where you feel comfortable being yourself. Sometimes, in our heaviest grief, it may be challenging to find a space that works for you because of the complexity of everything that is going on internally as you grieve and the lack of care in the external world. Try gentle walking if you cannot find a space that speaks to you, or you can come back to this exercise at a later time too.

For this exercise, what do you notice? Reflect on your authenticity creatively: by drawing a picture of yourself or writing a stream of consciousness. What are all the synonyms that describe you? What is it that makes you uniquely you?

In this safe space, imagine something you struggle with, such as difficult conversations or negative self-image challenges. Use what you created in the first part of the exercise to determine how to navigate these challenging situations with authenticity and hope. Apply these reflections to enhance your goal-attainment Hope Exercise from Chapter 11. How do these reflections get you closer to your goal?

Chapter 13

Maturing with Purpose

"I know for certain that we never lose the people we love, even to death...Their love leaves an indelible imprint in our memories. We find comfort by knowing that our lives have been enriched by having shared their love."

—Leo Buscaglia

With authenticity, we can be more purposeful about how we live, how we change, and thrive with intention and open heartedness.

After the losses, Lani wanted a roadmap to live in her purpose and continued with her goal-directed energy and meaning making. As she started to listen to herself more, she noticed shifts in her way of being—she felt lighter, she was more kind, and yet, she felt both more fragile and stronger. She explored these shifts through conversations, and she realized that she had a motivation to change from her prior way of being to her newly adapted way of being. Her motivation was to live a good life, inspired by new meaning making and perspective shifts. She knew she needed focused action to make this happen for herself, so she began consistently mapping out her intentions by asking herself, "How do I get closer, today, to the person I want to be?"

She focused on taking breaks throughout the day and responding to herself with kindness when she felt she was faltering. She had the support of her team: a few close friends, a therapist, and a coach. As she began living more intentionally, focused on how she wanted to feel each day and what she wanted to accomplish as a result, she got closer to her bigger life goal to make an impact in her community. Of course, she had missteps along the way and even days where she took big steps backwards, turning toward old ways of thinking about the world and herself. She stayed the course and fulfilled her goals with purpose.

As you continue to grow your authenticity, purpose roots out of that growth. In addition to authenticity, we may grow in purpose through inspiration, spiritual source, perspective shifting, and/or intentionality. These internal ways of being lead to inspired action and hopeful-living. They help keep you buoyant as you navigate injustices and criticisms of a dynamic world. I include in the following outline of how Lani's work is supported through a framework to develop purpose.

Brainstorming Framework for Making Change, Action Steps, and Strategies Work Example from Lani's Compounded Grief Experience – Instructions in Left Column and Lani's example responses in the right column.

Definition of Internal Shifts	Internal Shifts Example
• Perspective: Supported by reflection, you begin to make changes in your thinking and feeling patterns to take on new perspectives, ideas, and ways of being. Highlight some of your perspective shifts.	• Belief in self to try something outside of my comfort zone.
• Motivation: How you change and are encouraged through inspiration. This leads to increases in intrinsic motivation, the determination to do something different. What is your motivation for change?	• Motivated by wanting change, knowing that change may be difficult, and having the support of my grief support team to know that I can make mistakes, try new things, and not be attached to the outcome.
• Intentionality: Through focused action, we create spaces in our way of being to meet our desires and needs for internal shifts and motivation to take on a change. What can you do to be intentional about change?	• I must make the intentional time and space to continue exploring the fun, such as my concert going goal, and the service, such as giving back in the community.

Strategies

- Strategies: Brainstorm strategies that may be helpful for you, then select a few of those to try what may work best for your life.

- Repetition: Relies on the internal shifts to utilize strategies and shift old ways of thinking. How will you be sure repetition is part of your process?

Strategies

- During concert: Check in with myself three times to understand how I am feeling. Journal about this or simply note this in my mind. Ask how this relates to giving back in the community.

- Put a reminder on my calendar for three days after the concert to check in with myself. What did I learn about myself by trying something new? How can I use this information to follow through with my desire to serve the community?

- Repeat new self-discovery strategies and brainstorm ideas to do so. Next week I will try a new walking path.

Definition of External Conditions

- Community or human support: The people you are interdependent with and can rely on their support. Whom can you rely on for support?

- Structure: The intentional space, time, supports, and conditions you put in place to meet your needs and achieve your goals. How can you ensure you have space and time to achieve your goal(s)?

- Accountability: The community and structure that you rely on to create accountability systems that work for you. What will help you stay focused on your goal?

- Care for self: The conditions you put in place that increase your wellbeing. What is an example of care for yourself that relates to your goal?

External Conditions

- I want to talk to my friend and husband about the concert and how it went.

- I have made sure to create space in my days to ensure I am doing things that are in alignment with who I am becoming.

- Phone reminders help me with accountability. Journaling does too. So does telling my friend, husband, and grief support team about my goals.

- I will care for myself during this time by not overdoing things, taking time to rest, realizing change is a process, and prioritizing my self-development.

Take a moment to contemplate your goal from Chapter 11 and your reflection from Chapter 12 and engage with the coaching framework throughout this chapter to help make your next steps work for your individual needs. By focusing on your internal shifts, your specific strategies, and your network of support, you can live more purposefully and make your goals more attainable.

For your internal shifts, focus on your perspective by inquiring what you are feeling and thinking about yourself and others. What are you noticing about how your thoughts and feelings are changing? How can you be kinder to yourself and others?

For your motivation, find what works for you, and recognize that failure is inherent in this process. So is understanding your new way of being in the world. Ask yourself, what motivated you in the past to make a change? What has not worked for you? How has this shifted recently and what from your past can you rely on for motivation? What is the smallest factor you can use to consistently rely on for motivation?

Intentionality helps us live out our purpose by taking focused action, recovering when we make mistakes, and bringing us hope. Relearning your world means that you will make mistakes or missteps. Possibly more than you ever have before. That is okay. Do not let shame take hold in these moments. Lean into your authenticity and purpose and hold yourself with kindness as you reenter the world as a new person. Part of relearning the world is embracing mistakes and missteps, just as you would give grace to anyone recovering from any other injury. When I broke my wrist, it was easy to accept that I could not lift my cup of coffee the first few times I tried. In grief, I had to relearn so much more, and so of course my mistakes and missteps were much bigger than simply lifting a cup of coffee. I wish someone would have told me at the time that my shame had taken hold of what I had perceived as failures and let me know that this is part of the process as you become more decisive about how you live your life after loss. This is a hidden gift in grief and loss. We relearn our worlds to be more purposeful and in alignment with who we really are and who we are meant to be.

As you explore your authenticity and intentionality and notice your internal shifts, note all strategies that can help you meet your goal from the exercise at the end of the chapter. Pay attention to what your intuition and motivation tell you about each of them and select two to try. What do you notice about trying these strategies? Does one more naturally work for you? Use your intentionality to follow through with the strategies as often as you can for at least one week. Then extend that.

Finally, external conditions. External conditions include community and human support, both relational and tangible. These may cause you more pain or suffering or they may bring you more hope and contentment. If you are not finding the support that you want or need in these individuals or support services, keep trying to find what may work for you. What used to work for you may no longer work as you relearn your world, so be patient with yourself. Sometimes, you just need to have a direct conversation with someone that something is not working, and other times, you may not have the energy to do so in grief. You do not need to be the grief educator of others as you grieve, and you do want to find services that work for you. Also, structure, accountability, and care for self are part of the conditions for making shifts in your life. Consider, what can you do each day to ensure there is structure in your day to meet your goal? How will you hold yourself accountable for your shift? How will you care for yourself as you try to implement a new goal with clarity and purpose?

Chapter 13 Exercise

Build on your reflection from Chapter 12. Take time to get to know possibilities and yourself better with this framework.

Questions to ask for each section:
Internal Shifts

- What are you feeling and thinking about yourself and others?

- What are you noticing about how your thoughts and feelings are changing?

- How can you be kinder to yourself and others?

Strategies

- What has motivated you in the past to make a change?

- What has not worked for you?

- What is the smallest factor you can use to consistently rely on for motivation?

- What are one or two strategies you can start with?

- What do you notice about trying these strategies?

- Does one more naturally work for you?

External Conditions

- What can you do each day to ensure there is structure in your day to meet your goal?

- How will you hold yourself accountable for your shift?

- How will you care for yourself as you try to implement a new goal with intentionality?

Coaching Framework for Making Steps and Strategies Work – Your Example

Definition of Internal Shifts	Internal Shifts
• Perspective: Supported by reflection, you begin to make changes in your thinking and feeling patterns to take on new perspectives, ideas, and ways of being. Highlight some of your perspective shifts. • Motivation: How you change and are encouraged through inspiration. This leads to increases in intrinsic motivation, the determination to do something different. What is your motivation for change? • Intentionality: Through focused action, we create spaces in our way of being to meet our desires and needs for internal shifts and motivation to take on a change. What can you do to be intentional about change?	
Strategies	Strategies
• Strategies: Brainstorm strategies that may be helpful for you, then select a few of those to try what may work best for your life. • Repetition: Relies on the internal shifts to utilize strategies and shift old ways of thinking. How will you be sure repetition is part of your process?	

Definition of External Conditions	External Conditions
• Community or human support: The people you are interdependent with and can rely on their support. Whom can you rely on for support? • Structure: The intentional space, time, supports, and conditions you put in place to meet your needs and achieve your goals. How can you ensure you have space and time to achieve your goal(s)? • Accountability: The community and structure that you rely on to create accountability systems that work for you. What will help you stay focused on your goal? • Care for self: The conditions you put in place that increase your wellbeing. What is an example of care for yourself that relates to your goal?	

The Power of a Walk

I leave in the morning agitated and stressed,
My mind cannot get the word puzzles or consume the news or even
remember my cup of coffee.

I take a walk. The spring energies swirling,
The sun shining bright on me giving me life and hope.
Sometimes, that sun is just way too bright, though, and I retreat.

At times, I acknowledge it and do not have the energy to meet the sun or
the walk.
Today, I welcome it, and return home strengthened, renewed, and calm.

The word puzzles flow easily from my brain,
My heart opens to love,
And I remain in my power.

All because I took a walk.

Chapter 14

Living in Your Growth: Strategies for Continued Reflection, Nourishment, and Change

"The most beautiful people we have known are those who have known defeat, known suffering, known struggle, known loss, and have found their way out of the depths...Beautiful people do not just happen."

—Dr. Elisabeth Kübler-Ross

I wrote The Power of a Walk poem one morning after I reflected on my struggles and successes with my walking routine connected directly to my happiness. One of the hardest spaces in grief and loss to be in is learning to love yourself for who you are now, including all your flaws and strengths. Sometimes, this may require more intention from therapeutic and medicinal options too. Part of loving myself was focusing on happiness to root back into an innate personality characteristic of mine. The exercise I used the most to make this happen for myself was walking or running while expressing appreciation and owning up to my shame.

The combination of the BloomPath® with the strategies throughout the book may lead to a new way of living. Living in the in-between, which is present and aspirational, reflective and kind. It includes strategies, connection, reflection, being stuck, and adjusting.

While authoring this book, I was enrolled in a mindfulness modality course, and I was directed to look at my own baby picture and describe three attributes about myself in that picture. I chose kind, curious, and happy. I realized that I have been kind and curious, fostering both traits with care, but I have not really been intentionally happy in my life. Despite the optimistic nature of my innate personality traits, lived experiences have tempered my ability to access that happiness more consistently. As I continued to work through the course, I found more ways to root into myself by being reflective and determined about my happiness. This was not easy. Recognizing that happiness is a verb[18], I realized that I could be more focused on my happiness through my love of writing, creating, and movement while also holding space for critique and feeling the range of my emotions I needed to feel.

Working toward something with purpose and reflection is one way to build happiness. This is similar to how we explore grief. Healing is intentional and responsive, and it necessitates reflection. With this purpose, there is a level of practice involved that helps you get better at having the hard conversations, rooting into your emotions and not pushing them away. Embarking on this work is challenging, and it may cause points of pain or suffering because you are now awake in a way that is different, and that can be hard for you and the people around you. You are doing the hard work now, though, and if you push your grief aside without exploring healing, it may erupt in the future, potentially causing difficulty and frustration.

As you continue to focus on your goal and goal attainment strategies from previous chapters, consider small adjustments throughout your day to help you move closer to who you are and who you want to be while honoring the grieving that you want and need. You can hold space for despair and hope, anger and kindness, depression and contentment. It is okay and normal that challenging emotions and thoughts come up throughout the grieving process. Sometimes, despair is our best option as a response to a life changing event. Hold to these feelings with gentleness, and root back into your goodness, which is your ability to hold both the hard emotions and the hopeful ones. Walks help me root back into myself and grow my open-heartedness and compassion for myself. And the exercise from the mindfulness course that included me recognizing my innate traits from my baby picture gave me another way to access compassion for myself. This helped me explore the Identity Bloom to ground into these life-giving characteristics of mine.

Sometimes, all we can do is retreat, and other times, all we can do is fully live. So, what does it mean to whole-heartedly live and Bloom into yourself?

This is something that is not finite. Blooming has been happening all along your life journey and as you have engaged with the activities in this book. By making meaning, you can more fully appreciate who you are, where you have been, and where your life is headed. Consider what makes you thrive and who you want to be. These are tough, ongoing, adaptive, and responsive reflections. If people consistently knew the answers to these questions, the world would be different.

You can engage in Blooming into yourself in a way that's a little bit more outward, in a way that is buoyant and resolute. This can include bouncing ideas and frameworks about your thoughts and feelings from the internal to the external through engagement with others and reflection with yourself. This is living in between, in the paradox. The becoming that you are and the past that you were. With this determined confidence, we welcome growth and engage in connection. It is hard to hold a belief about yourself, about the world, about philosophies, without delving into those big questions with others so that you are not alone in your grief. And grief tends to bring up big questions and big feelings, and even sometimes, a new sense of loneliness that can both feel scary and create a pathway to open to hope.

While this chapter is all about living into yourself, I want to acknowledge the notion that we must Bloom into ourselves by living within and outward, making connections about our journeys, thoughts, and feelings, and connecting with other humans. Live inward by reflecting on your emotions, thoughts, and possibilities, or by practicing mindfulness, or engaging in a spiritual practice. And focus outward by engaging in those difficult conversations, sharing your talents, and practicing vulnerability. Connection and meaning making are a process.

Tending to the seeds of healing that you have planted and grown through this book not only includes active self-care such as fostering relationships, engaging in physical activity, and taking time to rest, but it also includes active reflective thought and feeling and tapping into yourself about lived grief, making connections to the past and present. Remember your brain is learning a new map[19] and relearning your world[20].

So how do you live while in the throes of grief, the ever-changing landscape that is your brain and your feelings and your experiences?

You are uniquely you because of your biology and your lived experiences that no one else has ever had or will ever have, because you are meant to live authentically. The work you have completed in this book helps you recognize your own individuality and how your individuality is shaped by your grief and loss—and universally all our worlds shaped through these experiences. Since you have been able to reflect on the holistic interactions of your grief and loss with your internal thoughts, emotions, and beliefs, external systems, and relationships and more, you now have your own individual compass to guide how you respond to and reflect on various losses in your life. We are constantly Blooming and pruning, growing and being stuck, being mindful and being reckless, and everything between these dichotomies. You exist in the in-between.

With your reflection, you Bloom by being your own north star and integrating the thirteen Blooms in your life that relate to your grief and loss, and you tend to those with care, honesty, and self-belief. You have the capacity to be your map by believing in yourself and who you are as a human, family member, friend, community member, and more amidst your brokenness. In the process of becoming, you are your north star. You navigate with love and believe in yourself.

As part of living whole-heartedly, being stuck is often part of the process. At many points in our lives sometimes we are simply stuck, whether that is stuck not meeting goals; stuck not having the hard conversations; stuck not believing in yourself; stuck in sorrow; stuck in depression, despair, and at those moments, it's okay to be stuck. Being stuck is still Blooming, and it is hard to see it in the moment, but in the months and years after, you may recognize how that stuck-ness led to even fuller Blooms and a more beautiful life. When I was in the hospital for a major depressive episode, I was in complete despair and utterly scared out of my mind about what this meant for me as a human here on Earth. How could anybody ever be a friend of mine in the future knowing this part of me? How could anybody trust me knowing that I have had these very painful and difficult moments? And how could anyone regard me as capable? These are all still painful questions for me that I grapple with regularly, and in those moments of being stuck, I was simply having to be. I can look back on those moments with a little more tenderness, a little more contentment, and understand that I have the capacity to heal continuously even when it feels like those moments have been a life sentence for chronic challenges related to deep pain and despair.

When I returned to work after the birth of my third daughter, five years after Evelyn's death, I was breastfeeding and working over fifty hours a week. While I may have appeared put together on the outside, I did not know that I was starting to spiral inward. Additionally, the pandemic hit, and we were grappling with the aftermath of the effects, sitting behind a screen in virtual meetings all day, every workday. The lack of sleep, my previous trauma, and my sedentary lifestyle all led to me stumbling once again with my mental health. Having experienced something similar before, I wanted so badly to force myself out of this stuck-ness, this pain. Of course, the more I tried to fight it, the more stuck I became.

Being stuck in life is like getting a vehicle stuck on a muddy country road. The more you fight it, the deeper your wheels turn into the mud and the more stuck you become. If you try to go too far backwards or too far forward, you are back to where you started from—stuck! And yet, if you move a little forward and a little backward, consistently, you will get unstuck (or eventually you will need to call for help and have someone help tow your vehicle out with their tractor).

Just as this example of a stuck car, as you are wholly living, try small adjustments and be gentle with yourself, accept that you are stuck and do not rush forward progress, and you will get to where you want to be. And when you are realizing you are stuck longer than you wished for, it may be worth calling in the "tow people" such as friends, family, and/or professionals to help you create movement in your life that speaks uniquely to you.

You may also consider where you are ambivalent in your life and how that is impacting you. If you find yourself in a loop of chronic contemplation without the change you want to manifest, be curious about how your ambivalence relates to your authenticity. Where is there dissonance? Is this something that you can tend to now or soon? I felt ambivalent about how I wanted to live my life five years ago. I did not make a change until after a year of processing my thoughts and feelings with my therapist and working on some internal shifts within my being. I had to explore a lot of my thinking and feeling before I felt ready to make a shift, and when I did make the shift, I still was not quite ready. One is never fully ready for a change they are making in their lives, but with support and understanding, you can make the small shifts that lead to the lifestyle changes you want to manifest. The promise of starting with small changes provides an opportunity to re-learn your world and who you are without being stuck in constant contemplation.

You have the BloomPath® for Grief and Loss; you have explored understanding your grief and engaging your paradox with your authenticity and purpose. Now, you have learned about living in the in-between and whole-heartedly and being stuck. You are an ever-changing being, and you deserve time to heal, rest, and discover. The roots of your grief bring new challenges and new understandings. New hopes and new fears. New loves and new dislikes. Wisdom that only you know. Remember, you exist in the in-between as a human broken-open to the possibilities of their life after loss and the depths of challenges as a griever. Root into your reflections, strategies, connection, stuck-ness, and small adjustments. Who are you becoming?

Chapter 14 Exercise

Revisit what you have completed from each chapter activity so far. What themes do you notice? Where are there gaps that you want to address? Where do you feel stuck?

Acknowledge your progress. What is that? Where do you feel the most hope?

Explore being stuck:

1. Which Internal Bloom(s) do you feel most stuck? How will you explore being stuck in these Blooms?

2. Which External Blooms(s) do you feel most stuck? How will you explore being stuck in these Blooms?

The Paradox of Grief Breaking Open

Grief draws me in and brings me out,
Shatters of new understanding
Lead me onto a pathway.

My soul feels the complexity and knows the levity,
As love opens me to the life that I am meant to live.

Challenged by new perspectives,
I honor my loss with compassion,
Surrendering to what was and what is to come.

The harbor unravels me anew.
I try on the new me.

My hope becomes something different,
As I take a path.
I Bloom out of open heartedness.

My mind awake with fresh ideas,
As wisdom leads me to the new life that I am meant to live.

Others help me take my path,
And bring me to new life.
Intention sets in, as I live in my purpose.

I embrace the journey,
Let grief unwind me free, and

Bloom into who I will be.

Chapter 15

Bloom

"Others want me to find closure. But closure is an illusion. There is no finality in loss. There are multiple beginnings and endings."

—Benjamin Allen

Bloom into who you are meant to be. As you continue to find movement and allow for stuck-ness within and for your grief, focus on how you integrate the BloomPath® and additional strategies in this book into your world and your life story. Grief exists beyond our minds, and it cannot be tied together to cure or fix. The BloomPath® helps you understand how thirteen different life factors can help you Bloom into your purpose and self-understanding by utilizing meaning making tools and hope-directed activities.

As a final reflection, tie the pieces of your story together. This is known as your denouement (dānoo'mäN), the French word that means untying and is used as the word that describes the end of a plot in which strands are tied together. Your denouement is suitable for the concept of in-between and paradox that have been included in this book. For the purpose of this chapter, denouement means to tie the pieces of your story together by making meaning about themes and the work from your exercises in this book and continue to tend to them, like a garden. Your own garden of purpose.

In the denouement for movies or theater productions, the pieces of the story are all brought together, and the matters, conflicts, and challenges are neatly explained or resolved. I like the word denouement because it fits when we think about ways to be more intentional about how we grow from reflecting on our past stories. With the BloomPath® you hold the capacity to look back at your experiences and your whole being in relationship to many facets of your life to better understand your grief and your denouement. The difference here, unlike in a movie or theater production, is that your journey will continue to unravel many denouements, and this is not tidy work. So, while you are circling in on a denouement right now, when you can engage and re-engage in these exercises in this book, a couple months or years down the road, you'll be able to continue to thread together a new denouement that is purposeful and integrates your wants and needs.

Writing this book has been a denouement for me. I have connected the dots of my early years, my interests and professional work, to my current years regarding my personal and professional life to write what has been in my heart and mind. Putting together the BloomPath® has been my cognitive, creative, and emotional Blooming into something much more than I was before. It has allowed me to explore more of my identity and spiritual development while bringing additional hope and healing into my life. Ten years ago, as I was sitting on the couch, alone in my home a few weeks after the death of my daughter, with nothing to do, nowhere to be, and falling, both swiftly and slowly into despair, I never would have thought that I would write this book and live all of the beautiful life experiences I have been fortunate to have since my daughter's death.

Part of the denouement for me is holding onto all the hope that has been brought into my life through connection, reflection, learning, curiosity, and open heartedness. While this is the denouement for my first ten years of healing, I enter the unknown for the next ten years, filled with more love and compassion for myself and others. As a teen, I was told to write is to think. But, to write is to feel and think. We have evolved to tend to our feelings rather than shut them off and ignore them. They play a significant part in our lives, and when those feelings are pushed aside or cut off from our ways of being to be more liked or to be more successful, we do others and ourselves a disservice.

For Lani's denouement, she continued to journal and find herself through music and spirituality while continuing the work on her marriage. She began to feel a bit more of a lightness a few years after the death of her dad, and she was grateful she took the time to be open and responsive to her grief needs. She continued to grieve her parents, and she celebrated and mourned their lives differently for the next couple of years. She was still sad about what she had lost in grief, and she was grateful for what she gained in her marital relationship and new friendships along with her newfound purpose helping others with their landscaping needs. She spent time exploring her health to hold both the grief and sadness with the newfound hope and renewal for her relationships. By focusing on her individual identity through spirituality and trying new things and rooting into the Professional Bloom as part of her purpose, she grew her confidence and understanding of herself and her grief needs. This helped her open up more fully and confidently in her marriage. Her husband grew his communication skills and found new life as well. He started to explore his grief more intentionally, and he started to love himself again, which he had not felt a steady level of contentment since the death of his parents many years ago.

As you continue to explore your grief and loss, one helpful way to tend to the seeds of your own Blooming is to go back through the BloomPath®. Check in with yourself about how you are doing in each of those Bloom areas. What are you grateful for? What can you do to reflect on these exercises after you complete reading this book? The end of this chapter provides you with an exercise to reflect. As you revisit the BloomPath®, pay attention to the shifting nature of each of the Blooms for you. What is the potential for you? In a few months, revisit Chapters 7 and 8 for the descriptions and questions to consider about each Bloom.

Continue to integrate the strategies from the book and live your life, as possibilities bring encouraging movement toward new goals and may also bring overwhelm because of the changes, newness, and frustrations about entering a new world. Were we meant to be firmly rooted or to be full of flight? Roots and Wings helps me hold both ends of the spectrum of life possibilities by rooting into myself, learning through the BloomPath® about my internal and external influences of grief and loss and my true authentic needs to create something meaningful in my life. If we are only rooted, we miss the possibilities of movement, learning new things, trying and tasting new experiences, and meeting other humans, wildlife, and natural experiences that help us grow into a Bloom that is bold, beautiful, and sturdy. If we are only in flight, we miss the possibilities of living into our journey, growing in community, and sticking around for all the seasons that also help us Bloom into ourselves, root into community, and connect with others.

To further integrate the lessons of this book into your life, consider writing a letter to yourself that reflects on your grief journey from the beginning of the book to its conclusion. What themes do you notice? What has given you life? What has been hard to navigate? What has challenged you and what has given you hope?

In this book, I provided several ways to interact with the BloomPath®. Your grief is continuing to be integrated as you continue to grow around it. As you grow to be a container for your grief, integrating your grief, you get bigger while the grief continues to take up space. This understanding is based on Tonkin's theory of 'growing around grief,' which suggests that the painful feelings remain present, but through new experiences, meeting others and the pursuit of new activities, enjoyment can be achieved[21]. With your growth, you may notice that tending to each of the Blooms more purposefully may not need as much support, and as you continue to grow, your Blooms will grow as an outflowing of your beauty and authenticity. The figure here illustrates Tonkin's concept of growing around grief.

You expand around your grief by continuing your growth while the loss is still there and a part of you.[22]

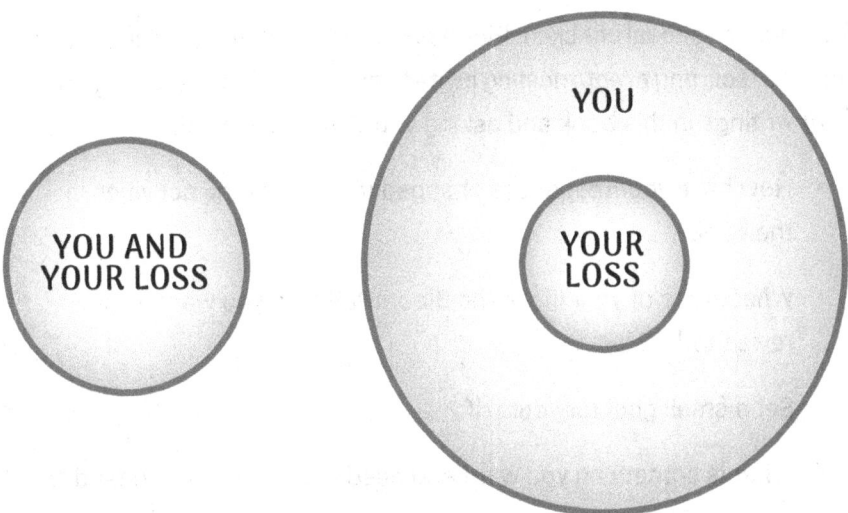

As you continue to navigate your own grief journey, know that all the missteps, the mistakes, the hurt, the challenges, and the resiliency are a part of your journey just as the hope, dreams, persistence, compassion, and progress are as well. You are a beautiful being meant to live your authentic life filled with an overflowing container of inspiration, love, and contentment. You have the capacity to call in loving kindness as you navigate the depths of your grief and loss.

Chapter 15 Exercise

Schedule an annual check-in. Pick a day and month, and put it in your calendar as a recurring event/meeting invite to check-in with yourself by revisiting your writings in this book and asking yourself a few questions:

- How have your responses changed to some of the activities in the book?

- What areas of your life in the BloomPath® do you want to revisit today?

- Set a small goal for yourself:

- What is something you want and need to do this week to tend to your grief?

    - How will you ensure you make this happen?

    - Whom can you talk to about this goal to gain support from an accountability partner to make this goal happen in your life?

- What have you noticed about yourself this year that you are curious about and want to keep developing?

No matter where you are on your grief journey, where you have been, and where you are right now, you are a vessel of strength. May your journey be filled with goodness and love. Kindness and compassion. And you, as a broken yet beautiful human being, living in your own authenticity and growing around your grief and losses to honor your presence, bravely live, integrate your experiences, and Bloom.

Acknowledgements

I am deeply grateful to my husband, Matt, whose unwavering support and encouragement have been a guiding light throughout this journey.

To my daughters, Evelyn, Madeleine, and Brielle, who are my greatest teachers and the deepest joys of my heart—thank you for the endless lessons in love and resilience that you offer me every day.

A heartfelt thank you to my editor, Kate Allyson. From our first meeting in graduate school to our reunion thirteen years later, I remain forever grateful for her friendship, guidance, and editorial acumen.

I also wish to extend my deepest thanks to the professionals and spiritual leaders who supported me through my grief and mental health challenges. Thank you to my friends and family who embrace my authenticity. And to all the teachers, professors, colleagues, and coaches who have shaped my path and helped me arrive here, I owe my sincerest appreciation.

About the Author

Eryn Elder, MA, is a certified grief and loss support specialist and an ICF-trained life coach and coach trainer who helps adults navigate the difficult journey of loss. Eryn is also the creator of the *BloomPath®*, a practical tool designed to help grievers find hope and start to heal authentically.

Through her one-on-one coaching, group sessions, workshops, and trainings, Eryn helps people rebuild their sense of self and purpose after loss. She co-hosts the podcast *Coaching as Benevolence*, where she shares thoughts on personal growth and living with compassion.

Eryn resides in Longmont, Colorado, with her husband and two children while honoring the memory of her first-born daughter.

Visit her website www.rootsandwingsgriefcoaching.com
Email Eryn eryn@rootsandwingsgriefcoaching.com
Follow Eryn on Facebook

Notes

1 (Centers for Disease Control and Prevention 2023)

2 (Friedman 2013)

3 (Kübler-Ross 1970)

4 (Williams 2015)

5 (Facing History & Ourselves 2021)

6 (O'Connor 2022), p. 9

7 (O'Connor 2022), p. 22

8 (The Mayo Clinic 2023)

9 (Williamson 2010)

10 (Jones 2024)

11 (O'Connor 2022)

12 (SUDC Foundation n.d.)

13 (Attig 1996)

14 (Cleveland Clinic 2022)

15 (Snyder 1994)

16 (Snyder 1991)

17 (Clear 2018)

18 (Pogosyan 2024)

19 (O'Connor 2022)

20 (Attig 1996)

21 (Tonkin 2009)

22 (Tonkin 2009)

References and
Further Reading

Attig, Thomas. 1996. *How We Grieve Relearning the World. Oxford University Press.*

C.R. Snyder, Lori M. Irving, and John R. Anderson. 1991. "Hope and Health." In *Handbook of Social and Clinical Psychology: The Health Perspective*, by C.R. Snyder and Donelson R. Forsyth, 285-305. Oxford: Pergamon Press.

Centers for Disease Control and Prevention. 2023. *Sudden Unexpected Infant Death and Sudden Infant Death Syndrome.* November 9. Accessed September 18, 2024. https://www.cdc.gov/sids/about/index.htm.

Clear, James. 2018. *Atomic Habits.* New York: Penguin Random House.

Cleveland Clinic. 2022. "What Ambiguous Loss Is and How to Deal with It." *Cleveland Clinic.* February 17. Accessed September 18, 2024. https://health.clevelandclinic.org/ambiguous-loss-and-grief.

Facing History & Ourselves. 2021. *Social Identity Wheel.* February 25. Accessed September 18, 2024. https://www.facinghistory.org/resource-library/social-identity-wheel.

Friedman, Russell. 2013. "Over 40 Life Experiences You Might Have That Cause You Grief." *The Grief Recovery Method.* March 1. Accessed September 18, 2024. https://www.griefrecoverymethod.com/blog/2013/03/over-40-life-experiences-you-might-have-cause-grief.

Kübler-Ross, Elisabeth. 1970. *On Death and Dying.* New York: MacMillan.

O'Connor, Mary Frances. 2022. *The Grieving Brain*. New York: HarperOne.

Pogosyan, Marianna. 2024. "3 Ideas from Aristotle on How to Build a Good LIfe." *Psychology Today*. May 8. Accessed September 18, 2024. https://www.psychologytoday.com/us/blog/between-cultures/202405/3-ideas-from-aristotle-on-how-to-build-a-good-life.

Sara Jones, Sara Albuquerque, and Patrícia M. Pascoal. 2024. "Grief and Sexual Intimacy: Exploring Therapists' Views of Bereaved Clients." *International Journal of Sexual Health* 425–437. doi:doi:10.1080/19317611.2024.2354815.

Snyder, C.R. 2000. *Handbook of Hope, Theory, Measures, and Applications*. San Diego: Academic Press

SUDC Foundation. n.d. *Sudden Unexpected Death Data Enhancement and Awareness Act*. Accessed September 18, 2024. https://sudc.org/legislation-and-policy/sudden-unexpected-death-data-enhancement-and-awareness-act/.

The Mayo Clinic. 2023. *Sudden Infant Death Syndrome (SIDS)*. July 19. Accessed September 18, 2024. https://www.mayoclinic.org/diseases-conditions/sudden-infant-death-syndrome/.

Tonkin, Lois. 2009. "Growing Around Grief - Another Way of Looking at Grief and Recovery." *Bereavement Care*, January 7: 10. doi:https://doi.org/10.1080/02682629608657376.

Williams, Lisa. 2015. "64 Myths About Grief that Just Need to STOP." *What's Your Grief*. August 4. Accessed September 18, 2024. https://whatsyourgrief.com/64-myths-about-grief-that-just-need-to-stop/.

Williamson, Marianne. 2010. *A Course in Weightloss*. Hay House, Inc.

www.ingramcontent.com/pod-product-compliance
Lightning Source LLC
Chambersburg PA
CBHW010936120626
46554CB00007B/2489